Kaposi's Sarcoma

Kaposi's Sarcoma

Pathophysiology and Clinical Management

edited by

John L. Ziegler
Veterans Administration Medical Center
and University of California
San Francisco, California

Ronald F. Dorfman
Stanford University Medical Center
Stanford, California

Marcel Dekker, Inc.   New York and Basel

Library of Congress Cataloging-in-Publication Data

Kaposi's sarcoma.

Includes index.
1. Kaposi's sarcoma. I. Ziegler, John L.
II. Dorfman, Ronald F. [DNLM: 1. Sarcoma,
Kaposi's. QZ 345 K165]
RC280.R4K36 1988 616.99'27 87-20089
ISBN 0-8247-7824-3

MARCEL DEKKER, INC.
270 Madison Avenue, New York, New York 10016

Current printing (last digit):
10 9 8 7 6 5 4 3 2 1

PRINTED IN THE UNITED STATES OF AMERICA

To Robert C. Frederes, with lasting gratitude

Preface

Kaposi's sarcoma has been an enigmatic neoplasm since its first description by Moritz Kaposi over 100 years ago. Until recently, its histogenesis has been controversial. Pathologists have argued whether the tumor is benign or malignant. The histologic picture is remarkably consistent despite a wide variety of clinical manifestations. Clinicians disagree over the optimal strategy for management. There is no uniform staging system. The sporadic occurrence of the tumor in older men of Eastern European origin and endemic forms of the tumor in Africa are a mystery. In the past two decades, the tumor has appeared increasingly in patients with iatrogenic immunosuppression and acquired immunodeficiency syndrome (AIDS).

The etiology of Kaposi's sarcoma has been attributed to genetic factors, cytomegalovirus, parasites, immunodeficiency, angiogenesis factors, and chemical carcinogens.

Kaposi's sarcoma provides an instructive model for multifactorial oncogenesis. This volume addresses the current etiology, pathophysiology, clinical features, and management of Kaposi's sarcoma. This comprehensive overview provides a current guide to clinical management and treatment, as well as a state-of-the-art compilation of etiology and pathogenesis. We hope the volume will be of particular interest to oncologists (especially physicians following the AIDS epidemic), pathologists, radiotherapists, dermatologists, and immunologists.

John L. Ziegler
Ronald F. Dorfman

Contents

Contributors

Jay H. Beckstead, M.D. Associate Professor, Department of Pathology, School of Medicine, University of California, San Francisco, California

Anthony M. Berson, M.D. Resident, Department of Radiation Oncology, School of Medicine, University of California, San Francisco, California

Ronald F. Dorfman, MB. Bch, FRC Path. Professor of Pathology and Co-Director of Surgical Pathology, Department of Pathology, Stanford University Medical Center, Stanford, California

W. Lawrence Drew, M.D., Ph.D. Director, Clinical Microbiology and Infectious Diseases, Mount Zion Hospital and Medical Center, San Francisco, California

John W. Harris, Ph.D., M.D.* Professor, Department of Radiation Oncology, School of Medicine, University of California, San Francisco, California

Eng-shang Huang, Ph.D. Professor, Departments of Medicine, Microbiology, and Immunology, Lineberger Cancer Research Center, University of North Carolina, Chapel Hill, North Carolina

---

**Current affiliation*: Medical Director, Department of Radiation Oncology, St. Joseph Hospital, Eureka, California.

Israel Penn, M.D. Professor, Department of Surgery, University of Cincinnati Medical Center, and Chief, Department of Surgery, Veterans Administration Medical Center, Cincinnati, Ohio

Teri A. Reed, M.D.* Resident, Department of Radiation Oncology, School of Medicine, University of California, San Francisco, California

Alexander C. Templeton, M.D. Professor, Department of Pathology, Rush Medical College, Presbyterian-St. Luke's Medical Center, Chicago, Illinois

Paul A. Volberding, M.D. Associate Professor, School of Medicine, University of California, and Chief, Medical Oncology and AIDS Activities Divisions, San Francisco General Hospital, San Francisco, California

Susan D. Wall, M.D. Assistant Chief, Department of Radiology, Veterans Administration Medical Center, and Assistant Professor, School of Medicine, University of California, San Francisco, California

William M. Wara, M.D. Professor and Vice Chairman, Department of Radiation Oncology, School of Medicine, University of California, San Francisco, California

Gary S. Wood, M.D. Assistant Professor, Departments of Dermatology and Pathology, Stanford University Medical Center, Stanford, California, and Chief, Department of Dermatology, Veterans Administration Medical Center, Palo Alto, California

John L. Ziegler, M.D. Associate Chief of Staff/Education, Veterans Administration Medical Center, and Professor, School of Medicine, University of California, San Francisco, California

---

**Current affiliation*: Assistant Professor, Department of Radiotherapy, Loyola University of Chicago, Stritch School of Medicine, Maywood, Illinois.

Kaposi's Sarcoma

1

Overview of Kaposi's Sarcoma: History, Epidemiology, and Biomedical Features

John L. Ziegler
Veterans Administration Medical Center
and University of California
San Francisco, California

Ronald F. Dorfman
Stanford University Medical Center
Stanford, California

HISTORY

Moritz Kohn was born on October 23, 1837, in the town of Kaposvár on the Kapos river in southern Hungary. After graduating from medical school in Vienna in 1861 he undertook postdoctoral training in surgery and obstetrics. Under the influence of his father-in-law, Professor Ferdinand Hebra, he entered the field of dermatology. In 1871, because of the number of other Kohns practicing in Vienna, he changed his surname to Kaposi, after his birthplace in Hungary (1).

The following year Kaposi published the famous paper on "idiopathic multiple pigmented sarcoma of the skin," a designation he later altered to "sarcoma idiopathicum multiplex hemorrhagicum" (2,3). He describes the characteristic nodules and plaques on the extremities in five men from his practice. As the illness progresses, edema develops and nodules appear on the face, trunk, and mucous membranes; some nodules ulcerate, but others regress spontaneously. In his initial cases death occurred in 2–3 years, but in a subsequent publication, he considers an indolent clinical course more characteristic (4). Regarding pathogenesis, Kaposi regards the tumor as multicentric in origin. He notes that "while it is quite possible that a carcinoma exists for a time locally and that a general carcinomatosis develops from it by metastasis, we must assume with regard to the present ailment that a general disease (dyscrasia) exists from the beginning" (2). He attributes the pigmentation to hemorrhage within the nodules, and likens the tumor to an angioma. This classic description was so distinctive as to merit the eponym "Kaposi's sarcoma" by Koebner (5).

EPIDEMIOLOGY

Classic Kaposi's Sarcoma

Increments of knowledge about Kaposi's sarcoma have accumulated over four distinct periods (6). Until the 1950s, Kaposi's sarcoma was considered a rare disease, confined largely to episodic occurrences in individuals who originated from Eastern Europe, Poland, Italy, and Russia. The most comprehensive collection of cases was reported in a monograph by Samuel Bluefarb in 1957 (3). In the "classic," sporadic cases, the male-female ratio is as high as 17:1, with the majority occurring in the fifth through ninth decades of life.

Although geographic predisposition is evident, familial cases are distinctly rare (7). Bluefarb disputed the impression that Kaposi's sarcoma is limited almost exclusively to Jews, citing multiple reports of non-Jewish patients in Italy, Poland, and Russia. Since immigrants from "endemic" areas in the United States are more prone to Kaposi's sarcoma, it is likely that they carry a genetic susceptibility to the disease (8). Rare, atypical cases were reported in children and blacks.

The second period of important epidemiologic observations took place in the late 1950s and 1960s in tropical Africa. With the establishment of medical schools and cancer registries, Kaposi's sarcoma emerged as a very common neoplasm. An extensive study in Uganda showed Kaposi's sarcoma to comprise 8.7% of malignant tumors in males (as opposed to 0.6% in females). The incidence rose steadily after the third decade (9). The largest series was collected by Oettlé and Lothe, published in the proceedings of a symposium held in Kampala, Uganda, in 1961 (10). Although the precise geographic distribution has not been mapped out in Africa, the disease tends to predominate in Eastern Zaire, Rwanda, Burundi, and Western Uganda and diminishes in incidence as one travels north, south, east, and west (9,11, 12).

Kaposi's Sarcoma in Africa

As opposed to the apparent ethnic determinants in classic Kaposi's sarcoma, the disease in Africans tends to be more determined by geography. Population migrations in the western Rift Valley have resulted in a broad mix of tribal groups of Nilotic, Sudanic, Bantu, and Nilo-Hamitic origins. There is no obvious tribal predisposition to Kaposi's sarcoma, but tribal and geographic factors are confounding in epidemiologic analyses in Africa. No cases of Kaposi's sarcoma in non-Africans were reported in Uganda among 340 patients observed over a 5-year period, whereas 4 cases would be expected on a population basis (11). Although reported occasionally in Eskimos, Kaposi's sarcoma is extremely rare in Asians, Orientals, Arabs, and non-African blacks (12). Unlike the distribution of Burkitt's lymphoma, the demographic features of Kaposi's sarcoma bear no relationship to the endemicity of malaria. Despite the knowledge of geographic determinants of Kaposi's sarcoma in Africa, there are no clues as to environmental or genetic predisposing factors.

Careful studies of African cases have disclosed clinical variants that were not described in the classic cases (13). Although the typical "nodular" form was most common, this was observed in some patients to progress locally to a more "sarcomatous" or "florid" form. An "infiltrative," deeply invasive form was also noted. Finally, Kaposi's sarcoma in childhood was predominantly "lymphadenopathic" and had a rapid downhill course. These clinical variants correlated to some extent with histologic changes that indicated tumor cell morphological evolution.

Kaposi's Sarcoma and Immunodeficiency

The third phase of epidemiologic observations took place in the 1970s, when unexpected numbers of cases of Kaposi's sarcoma were observed among organ transplant recipients and in other conditions associated with iatrogenic immunosuppression. Kaposi's sarcoma usually developed about 1–2 years after immunosuppressive treatment was begun. In contrast to the classic form, the male-female ratio was about 2:1, with about one-quarter of the patients under 40 years of age. An unusual feature was the tendency for some tumors to regress spontaneously when immunosuppressive treatment was reduced or stopped (14). The association of Kaposi's sarcoma and immunosuppression is discussed in detail in Chapter 5.

Kaposi's Sarcoma and AIDS

The marked association of Kaposi's sarcoma with the current epidemic of acquired immunodeficiency syndrome (AIDS) comprises the fourth and most recent phase of epidemiologic study. Although indistinguishable histologically from classic lesions, Kaposi's sarcoma in AIDS varies from single, localized lesions to widespread cutaneous and visceral involvement. Interestingly, when Kaposi's sarcoma occurs in an African with AIDS, the disease is atypically aggressive when compared with the endemic form (15). Epidemiologic studies in the United States and Europe show that Kaposi's sarcoma predominates in homosexual men, accounting for about 50% of AIDS cases. Although reported in other risk groups, the tumor is distinctly uncommon: only 4% of intravenous drug abusers with AIDS develop Kaposi's sarcoma (16). On rare occasions, homosexual men are reported to develop Kaposi's sarcoma in the absence of infection by human immunodeficiency virus (HIV) (17). These observations point to additional cofactors, unique to homosexual men, that predispose to Kaposi's sarcoma.

Summary

To summarize, the epidemiology of Kaposi's sarcoma has raised many more questions than answers. Its sporadic, worldwide occurrence, predominating in men of certain ethnic origins, implies genetic and possibly hormonal determinants. The high frequency of the tumor in various tribal groups residing in eastern and central Africa suggests environmental influences. The unusual geographic coincidence of epidemicity in an area where Kaposi's sarcoma was already endemic (i.e., central and eastern Africa) invites speculation about a common link, such as another sexually transmitted disease, insect vectors, or animal reservoirs. Although patients with endemic Kaposi's sarcoma are seronegative for HIV (18), another associative connection between the two conditions may exist. The development of the tumor in immunosuppressed individuals points to a relationship of Kaposi's sarcoma to the immune system. Taken together, these features indicate a multifactorial etiology that involves a complex interaction among genetic predisposition, immune perturbations, and environmental factors. Thus, the pathogenesis of Kaposi's sarcoma becomes a fascinating paradigm for dissecting the causes of neoplasia.

BIOLOGIC FEATURES

After decades of controversy, the weight of evidence points to the endothelium as the progenitor cell of Kaposi's sarcoma. Recent studies, detailed in Chapter 3, implicate lymphatic endothelium as the tissue of origin, but the presence of abortive capillaries and extravasated erythrocytes leaves lingering questions as to the participation of blood vascular endothelium. Some workers, with good reason, have proposed that Kaposi's sarcoma is not a true "neoplasm" but is a generalized endothelial proliferative disorder, similar generically to the multifocal lymphoproliferation seen in infectious mononucleosis (19,20).

Kaposi's sarcoma does not behave like other soft tissue sarcomas, which grow locally and metastasize eventually to other organs. In its earliest stages it has the benign appearance of granulation tissue or stasis dermatitis. In AIDS patients, minute foci of Kaposi's sarcoma can be detected in the lymph node capsule and sinusoids, often accompanied by angioproliferation elsewhere in the node (19,21). Thus, one could argue the existence of "pre-Kaposi" lesions, consisting simply of multiple foci of hyperplastic endothelium. Over time and with the probable confluence of other factors, localized endothelial proliferative lesions develop into the more characteristic spindle cell appearance of Kaposi's sarcoma and then evolve clonally into a more malignant phenotype. The variations in histologic and clinical morphology suggest that the progenitor cell is multipotential and can manifest tumors with the characteristics of a variety of mesenchymal neoplasms (12).

PATHOGENESIS

The anatomic predilection of cutaneous Kaposi's sarcoma for the extremities, sites of previous trauma, and a tendency toward symmetry along lines of cleavage has led to considerable speculation regarding pathogenesis. The atypical behavior of the neoplasm in children, women, and immune-compromised individuals provides grounds for speculation about systemic hormonal or immune influences on tumor appearance and growth. In these cases, the tumor is far more aggressive, with multiple sites of involvement of every visceral organ (22). Rare instances of involvement of the brain by Kaposi's sarcoma in patients with AIDS (23) suggests the ability of these tumors to metastasize in the advanced stages, since the brain is devoid of lymphatic endothelium and is an unlikely source of "primary" Kaposi's sarcoma. The clinical variants of Kaposi's sarcoma and the natural history of tumor evolution (e.g., the progression of patch-stage lesions to plaques and of nodules to florid tumors) is consistent with clonal progression of the malignant phenotype over time.

The many theories of the pathogenesis of Kaposi's sarcoma are diverse and fall into five broad categories: (1) genetic predisposition; (2) a role for an infectious agent; (3) a general systemic influence of hormonal, neural, or vascular factors; (4) a manifestation of a generalized reticuloendothelial system disorder; and (5) the action of a systemic carcinogen on vascular tissues (3). These hypotheses are each supported by a variety of observations, summarized in Table 1.

Genetic Factors

Epidemiologic evidence argues for a genetic predisposition to Kaposi's sarcoma, but there are few supporting data from the laboratory. Chromosome analysis must be undertaken on tumor tissue in culture, and to date there is no convincing report of Kaposi's sarcoma growing in vitro. Genetic marker research is limited to

Table 1 Factors in the Pathogenesis of Kaposi's Sarcoma

Factors	Supporting observations
Genetic factors	
Hormonal	High prevalence in men
Immunoregulatory	HLA-DR association
Ethnic	Common among Jews and immigrants from Eastern Europe
Infection	
Cytomegalovirus (CMV)	CMV DNA found in some tumors; high seroprevalence in susceptible populations; cytomegalovirus carries cell-transforming genes
Other agent (?)	Geographic endemicity in Africa
Systemic effect	
Hormonal	High prevalence in men; spontaneous regression
Neural	Symmetrical distribution; predilection for sites of previous trauma
Vascular	Endothelial origin
Reticuloendothelial disorder	
Impaired immune "surveillance"	High incidence in immune-suppressed patients; spontaneous regressions
Immune dysregulation	Angioproliferative lesions in some patients; association with other lymphoproliferative disorders
Circulating carcinogen	
Nitrite abuse	Significant association in AIDS
Environmental carcinogens	Plastic (polyvinyl) products stimulate vasogenic tumors

prevalence studies of histocompatibility antigens. These demonstrate a two- to threefold excess of HLA-DR5 expression and a slightly reduced frequency of HLA-DR3 expression both in AIDS-associated and in classic Kaposi's sarcoma (24,25). A recent study also associates HLA-B35 frequency with the development of AIDS in Italian patients and confirms the DR5 linkage to Kaposi's sarcoma (26). There has been some technical difficulty in HLA phenotyping of patients with AIDS-related complex (ARC) and AIDS because of the presence of lymphotropic antibody. The antigens HLA-DR3 and DR5 are associated with other autoimmune diseases and may confer a general susceptibility to AIDS independent of Kaposi's sarcoma (27–30).

These genetic markers may be linked to immune response genes that modulate or impair the immune response, or their own specific configuration may modify their function as accessory molecules in antigen presentation and recognition. The latter hypothesis gains support from the observation that monoclonal antibodies directed against the specific HLA-DR gene products alleviate the associated autoimmune disorder in animal models (28). Unfortunately, most immune disorders linked to specific HLA genotypes are not all-or-none associations, giving rise to a polygenic theory of disease susceptibility (27). Further, histocompatibility genes have hypervariable alleles, permitting a high degree of polymorphism. A new technique that takes advantage of restriction fragment length polymorphism has refined the HLA-disease associations and should be applied to population studies of Kaposi's sarcoma (31).

Another consideration of genetic predisposition involves the male predominance of Kaposi's sarcoma. Are there male-associated factors (e.g., hormonal) that are predisposing? Conversely, are there female determinants that are protective? Certainly, the tumor in women (particularly in pregnancy) is far more agressive than in men, although in children there are no clinical differences in boys or girls. Treatment with estrogen in a few isolated instances has not altered tumor behavior (32). There are subtle differences in immunity and vascular reactivity in men and women, but these seem unlikely explanations.

Finally, the apparent genetic influences may be explained by a vertically transmitted virus that affects the endothelium. A fascinating animal model was reported by Lacey and colleagues in which a bovine papilloma virus containing an extra copy of the transforming gene region was introduced via a plasmid vector into the germ cells of mice (33). These transgeneic mice develop multifocal dermatofibromas after a latent period of 6–7 months. The tumors are initially benign but become malignant and locally invasive, appearing predominantly in sites of trauma. The authors suggest that this model of genetic predisposition requires additional oncogenic events to induce the full malignant phenotype. These may involve exposure to viruses, carcinogens, or growth factors. The parallels of this model to Kaposi's sarcoma are provocative.

Infectious Agent

A role of infection in Kaposi's sarcoma has long been sought. The only putative agent thus far is cytomegalovirus, first identified by Giraldo and colleagues in biopsy cultures from African patients in 1972 (34). The accumulated evidence over the past 15 years continues to implicate cytomegalovirus as a potential cofactor, but a direct, oncogenic role is unlikely (reviewed extensively in Chapter 4). The existence of another viral agent is still possible. In AIDS patients, HIV has not been identified in tumor lesions by molecular localization techniques (35) but there is one report of the observation of a retrovirus in Kaposi's sarcoma by electron microscopy (36). With the resurgence of interest in Kaposi's sarcoma as a manifestation of AIDS, it is possible that an "infectious" etiologic agent will be discovered.

Systemic Influences

The possibility of systemic influences on the genesis and behavior of Kaposi's sarcoma has long been entertained. The implications of a lymphatic endothelial origin point to the influence of oncogenic substances in the lymphatic circulation. Because of the relatively high incidence of spontaneous regression, one hypothesis holds that the tumors respond to humoral substances reminiscent of hormone-responsive tumors (37). Chapter 6 explores this proposal further.

A final speculation in this category concerns a role for neural factors. Lymph nodes and lymphatic endothelium receive autonomic innervation, but little is known of neurotransmittors and neuroendothelial interaction. The local release of neurally derived vasogenic transmittors could influence the proliferative state of the endothelium in a paracrine fashion (38). This possibility has never been explored in relation to neoplasia, but there are indications that local neurotropic substances, unrelated to nerve impulses and neurotransmitters, can augment biologic responses such as calcium metabolism, embryonal development, blastema formation, organ regeneration, and immune responses (39). Thus, research into neurotropic factors may reveal how local anatomic events can influence the development and growth of Kaposi's sarcoma.

Reticuloendothelial Disorder

The relationship of Kaposi's sarcoma to the immune system is still unresolved. Common features can be summarized as follows. (1) The tumor emerges in immunosuppressed individuals (see Chapter 5). (2) About one-third of patients with Kaposi's sarcoma had or developed second malignancies, over half of which were of lymphoreticular origin (40). Some of these cases involve the appearance of "collision" tumors in which Kaposi's sarcoma and lymphoma appear side by side (41,42). (3) Kaposi's sarcoma is associated with other diseases that reflect perturbation of immunity, such as leprosy, tuberculosis, diabetes mellitus, malabsorption, systemic lupus erythematosus, polymyositis, and aplastic anemia (6,8,9,14). (4) There is evidence of tumor-associated antigens and tumor-directed impairment of cutaneous delayed hypersensitivity (43,44). (5) There is a close histologic resemblance of early Kaposi's sarcoma to an inflammatory response, with participation of lymphocytes, plasma cells, and macrophages (12). (6) There is common involvement of lymph nodes by the tumor (45).

The relationship of Kaposi's sarcoma to the reticuloendothelial system can be better understood in light of the immune system of the skin (46). This is viewed to be in dynamic equilibrium with lymphoid organs. The element of commonality is the participation of the endothelial cell in the immune and inflammatory responses. The ability to express Ia antigens and to present new antigens to immune cells places the endothelial cell at a critical juncture in the immune response (47). Following injury, endothelial cells express C3b and Fc receptors (48). We can infer from these important functional roles that the endothelial cell also responds to systemic and local immunoregulatory signals that augment or suppress immune responses.

The intriguing relationship of Kaposi's sarcoma to immune events prompted Warner and O'Loughlin to postulate that the tumor is a "by-product" of a local graft-versus-host reaction, mediated by activation of an oncogenic virus and by liberation of angiogenic factors from stimulated lymphoid cells (49). In support of this contention is the observation of an unexpected number of tumors in recipients of poorly matched as opposed to well-matched donor kidneys (50). Others have postulated that Kaposi's sarcoma derives from lymphoid "stimulation" in a setting in which the immune system is actively compensating or is dysregulated; the stimulating agents are suggested to be angiogenic lymphokines (37). This hypothesis is developed more fully in Chapter 6.

A final consideration is the "immune surveillance" hypothesis, which proposes immune elimination of nascent tumors by recognition of tumor-associated antigens. It is clear that "tumor immunity" is a demonstrable phenomenon that involves both natural [e.g., natural killer cell and lymphocyte-activated killer (LAK) cell] and adaptive (e.g., specific cytotoxic T cell) mechanisms. Tumors may exhibit neoantigens of embryonal or viral origin or may alter their surface expression of histocompatibility antigens (51). Thus, one may specualte that Kaposi's sarcoma begins as benign endothelial proliferations that "escape" local immune recognition and grow as autonomous, multifocal tumors. Evidence in favor of this mechanism includes the presence of immune and inflammatory cells within the tumor, the observation of spontaneous regression, the finding of tumor-associated antigens that mediate a delayed hypersensitivity response, and the regression of tumors associated with topical immune stimulants or reduction of immunosuppressive medication. Tumors develop a variety of mechanisms to escape immune detection. A principal role is assigned to major histocompatibility (MHC) antigens, which are often altered during oncogenesis. For example, in an adenovirus-12 mouse tumor model in which class I MHC antigens are suppressed, Tanaka and colleagues were able to induce immune detection and elimination of tumors by transfecting the tumor cells with class I MHC genes (52). Although other mechanisms influence tumor rejection, the possibility of altered histocompatibility antigens in Kaposi's sarcoma warrants study.

Systemic Carcinogen

McCarthy and Pack first drew attention to the possibility that a systemic carcinogen was acting on the vascular tissue, perhaps accounting for the bilateral and symmetrical distribution of Kaposi's sarcoma (53). A number of candidate agents can cause endothelial hyperplasia and neoplasia, including azo compounds, vinyl chloride, and methylhydrazine derivatives (54–58). A systematic search for potential carcinogenic substances has not been undertaken in Kaposi's sarcoma, nor are there persuasive epidemiologic clues that implicate environmental exposure to carcinogens. The only potential candidate surfaced in studies of AIDS-associated Kaposi's sarcoma, in which "recreational" exposure to nitrite inhalants was significantly associated with Kaposi's sarcoma (59,60). Nitrites have carcinogenic potential by virtue of endogenous N-nitrosation reactions that produce mutagenic and carcinogenic N-nitroso derivatives (55). The "nitrite connection" in AIDS-associated Kaposi's sarcoma is compounded because nitrite use is another marker of sexual promiscuity that predisposes independently to AIDS (61). Further, although nitrite ingestion has been linked with gastric cancer in Japan, an inverse relationship was found in an epidemiologic study in Britain (62). Alternatively, amyl nitrite may exert its effects indirectly by altering immune responses (63). It remains possible that carcinogens are perhaps one of several factors that can induce Kaposi's sarcoma.

IMPLICATIONS FOR THERAPY

Kaposi's sarcoma is a relatively well differentiated tumor with a very low growth fraction (64). Despite its indolent clinical behavior the tumor is remarkably responsive to irradiation and chemotherapy (see Chapters 9 and 10). The reason for this may lie in the wide range of potential tumor doubling times (10–200 days) and to high rates of cell loss (64). In mixed cellularity Kaposi's sarcoma, the vascular component appears more sensitive to chemotherapy than the spindle cell component, showing additional evidence of tumor heterogeneity (9). Clinically, the nodular lesions respond well to radiation therapy (Chapter 9) and to chronic alkylating agent treatment. The more sarcomatous and lymphadenopathic tumors respond to therapy with vinca alkyloids, dacarbazine, actinomycin D, doxorubicin, bleomycin, and nitrosoureas administered singly and in various combinations (Chapter 10). The growth characteristics and treatment responses of Kaposi's sarcoma are very similar to those of Hodgkin's disease.

It is now apparent that successful management of Kaposi's sarcoma in immunosuppressed patients will involve restoration of immune function. As discussed above, it is not clear whether this host determinant reflects a tumor-directed immune response or another immune-mediated regulatory process. Any forms of potential "immunotherapy" of Kaposi's sarcoma must discriminate between these two possibilities.

Newer approaches to cancer treatment involve concepts of "biotherapy" that employ natural, growth-inhibiting substances. Such approaches in Kaposi's sarcoma find fertile soil. Already, treatment with interferons has produced tumor responses that compete with those achieved by chemotherapy (65). Another lymphokine, tumor necrosis factor, is highly toxic to endothelial cells and may prove to be a useful agent (66).

Many tumors retain some of the phenotypic and functional characteristics of their progenitor cell. Kaposi's sarcoma displays features suggestive of its endothelial origin, such as production of prostaglandins, synthesis of fibronectin and type IV collagen, and expression of endothelial antigens (see Chapters 3 and 6) (67). Since endothelial cells are responsible for capillary transport, regulation of plasma lipid, maintenance of hemostasis, and other important functions (68,69), we must assume that these characteristics may be found in Kaposi's sarcoma tissue. Further, it is logical to assume that neoplastic endothelium will respond to the normal regulatory signals that influence endothelial function. Thus, further research into the biology of Kaposi's sarcoma may disclose regulatory molecules (e.g., inhibitors of angiogenesis) that will modulate the behavior of the neoplasm.

SUMMARY

Kaposi's sarcoma is a thoroughly enigmatic condition with protean clinical manifestations and an obviously multifactorial etiology; sorting out the sequence of pathogenetic events is a major challenge for the experimental oncologist. Oncogenesis is best understood as a stepwise phenomenon. Experimentally, three events—initiation, promotion, and progression—are recognized (55). Initiation involves the alteration of DNA by a chemical, physical or biologic agent that confers malignant potential onto the cell genotype. Promotion involves the action of agents that alter the expression of genetic information in the cell. Progression is recognized as the clonal evolution of established tumors that accounts for heterogeneity and varied phenotypic manifestations (70). New knowledge regarding the action of "oncogenes" (71,72) indicates that proto-oncogenes (genes that are associated with cell transformation but are constitutively silent) can become activated by a variety of deregulatory or mutational events. Cooperating families of oncogenes, activated over time, then direct the cell toward a malignant phenotype. Genetic instability and environmental pressures (e.g., chemotherapy) are responsible for continued phenotypic evolution of the growing tumor.

One of the challenges in the genesis of Kaposi's sarcoma is to learn more of the interface between the genetic, environmental, and immune factors (Figure 1) in search of a unifying hypothesis. Perhaps the simplest general explanation is that an inherited genetic predisposition influences the immune response, which, when

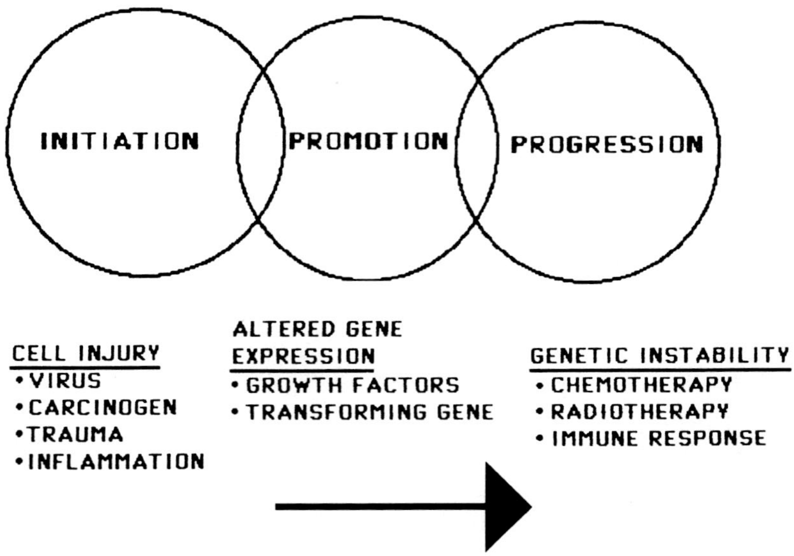

Figure 1 Pathogenesis of Kaposi's sarcoma is viewed as a continuous process of interlocking phases over time. The initial injury (e.g., cytomegalovirus infection of endothelial cells) perturbs cellular DNA. A second event (e.g., activation of transforming oncogene or influence of angiogenic growth factors) may alter or augment gene expression, leading to cell transformation. Intrinsic genetic instability of the malignant cell can lead to clonal evolution of the neoplastic phenotype.

stimulated, preferentially promotes endothelial hyperplasia. Individuals with this genetically controlled predisposition develop Kaposi's sarcoma only in multifocal endothelial cells that have been "initiated" previously by virus, carcinogen, or injury. As hyperplasia persists, additional "promoting" substances may provoke transformation. Alternatively, lack of inhibitory stimuli or alterations in cellular receptors for regulatory substances play a role in progression. The recent discovery of a transforming gene in Kaposi's sarcoma DNA provides evidence for the neoplastic state of the tumor once it is detectable clinically (73).

As the major interface between the tissues and the lymphatic and blood vascular capillary circulation, the endothelium is continually exposed to circulating viruses and carcinogens and to local trauma and inflammation. Thus, a variety of potential initiating and promoting insults can impinge on endothelial cells. This variety may partially explain how a single tissue could become neoplastic under widely disparate epidemiologic circumstances. Once damaged (e.g., by virus, such as cytomegalovirus, by nitrites or other circulating carcinogen, or by other substances entering the lymphatic circulation), initiated endothelial cells await the arrival of local or systemic "promoting" substances that induce the neoplastic change.

RECENT DEVELOPMENTS

AIDS-associated Kaposi's sarcoma was studied for the presence of HIV-DNA sequences and for chromosomal abnormalities (74). None of 13 tissue samples disclosed evidence of HIV sequences in DNA. Further, none had hepatitis B virus (HBV) sequences and only two had cytomegalovirus (CMV) sequences. Both of the latter patients had generalized CMV infection. Short-term cell cultures of Kaposi's sarcoma displayed endothelial markers and chromosomal rearrangements that were monoclonal in the same culture. These rearrangements varied from culture to culture and even in cultures from the same biopsy. This important study shows that HIV, HBV, and CMV are not related directly to the oncogenesis of Kaposi's sarcoma, and that this neoplasm contains chromosomal rearrangements that indicate its polyclonal nature.

REFERENCES

1. Braun M. Classics in oncology. Moritz Kaposi, M.D. CA 1982; 32:340–1.
2. Kaposi M. Classics in oncology. Idiopathic multiple pigmented sarcoma of the skin. CA 1982; 32:342–7 (translated from the original German from Arch Dermatol Syph [Berlin] 1872; 4:265–73).
3. Bluefarb S. Kaposi's sarcoma. In: Multiple Idiopathic Hemorrhagic Sarcoma. Springfield, Illinois, Charles C Thomas, 1957.
4. Kaposi M. Zur nomenclatur des idiopathischen pigmentsarkom Kaposi. Arch Dermatol Syph (Berlin) 1894; 29:164.
5. Koebner H. Kranken vorstellung (idiopathisches multiples sarcoma hemorrhagicum der extremitaten). Arch Dermatol Syph (Berlin) 1909; 94:121.
6. Ziegler JL, Templeton AC, Vogel CL. Kaposi's sarcoma. A comparison of classical, endemic and epidemic forms. Semin Oncol 1984; 11:47–52.
7. DiGiovanna JJ, Safai B. Kaposi's sarcoma. Retrospective study of 90 cases with particular emphasis on the familial occurrence, ethnic background and prevalence of other diseases. Am J Med 1981; 71:779–83.
8. Laor Y, Schwartz RA. Epidemiologic aspects of Kaposi's sarcoma. J Surg Oncol 1979; 12:299–303.
9. Templeton AC. Tumors in a Tropical Country. Berlin, Springer-Verlag, 1973.
10. Ackerman LV, Murray JF. Symposium on Kaposi's sarcoma. Basel, S. Karger, 1963.
11. Taylor JF, Smith PG, Bull D, Pike MC. Kaposi's sarcoma in Uganda: geographic and ethnic distribution. Br J Cancer 1972; 26:483–97.
12. Templeton AC. Kaposi's sarcoma. Pathol Annu 1981; 16:315–36.
13. Taylor JF, Templeton AC, Vogel CL, et al. Kaposi's sarcoma in Uganda: a clinico-pathological study. Int J Cancer 1971; 8:122–35.
14. Harwood AR, Osoba D, Hofstader SL, et al. Kaposi's sarcoma in recipients of renal transplants. Am J Med 1979; 67:759–65.

15. Bayley AC. Aggressive Kaposi's sarcoma in Zambia, 1983. Lancet 1984; 1:1318–20.
16. Desjarlais DC, Marmor M, Thomas P, Chamberland M, Zolla-Pazner S, Spencer DJ. Kaposi's sarcoma among four different risk groups. N Engl J Med 1984; 310:1119 (letter).
17. Afrasiabi R, Mitsayasu R, Nishanian P, Schwartz K, Fahey JL. Characterization of a distinct subgroup of high risk individuals with Kaposi's sarcoma who present with normal T-cell number and T4:T8 ratio and negative HTLV-III/LAV serology (abstract). Proc ASCO 1986; 5:2.
18. Biggar RJ, Melbye M, Kestems I, et al. Kaposi's sarcoma in Zaire is not associated with HTLV-III infection (letter). N Engl J Med 1984; 311:1051.
19. Costa J, Rabson AS. Generalized Kaposi's sarcoma is not a neoplasm (letter). Lancet 1983; 1:58.
20. Brooks JL. Hypothesis. Kaposi's sarcoma: a reversible hyperplasia. Lancet 1986; 2:1309–11.
21. Harris NL. Hypervascular follicular hyperplasia and Kaposi's sarcoma in patients at risk for AIDS. N Engl J Med 1984; 310:462–3 (letter).
22. Friedman-Kien AE, Laubenstein LJ, Rubenstein P, et al. Disseminated Kaposi's sarcoma in homosexual men. Ann Intern Med 1982; 46:693–700.
23. Levy RM, Bredesen DE, Rosenblum ML. Neurological manifestations of the acquired immunodeficiency syndrome (AIDS). Experience at UCSF and review of the literature. J Neurosurg 1985; 62:475–98.
24. Pollack MS, Safai B, Myskowski PI, Gold JWM, Dupont B. Frequency of HLA and GM immunogenetic Kaposi's sarcoma. Tissue Antigens 1983; 21:1–8.
25. Contu L, Cerimele D, Carcassi C, et al. Immunogenetic and immunologic study on classic Kaposi's sarcoma. IRCS Med Sci 1984; 12:891–2.
26. Smeraldi RS, Fabio G, Lazzarin A, et al. HLA-associated susceptibility to acquired immunodeficiency syndrome in Italian patients with human-immunodeficiency virus infection. Lancet 1986; 2: 1187–9.
27. Shoenfeld Y, Schwartz RS. Immunologic and genetic factors in autoimmune diseases. N Engl J Med 1984; 311:1019–29.

28. McDevitt HO. The molecular basis of autoimmunity. Clin Res 1985; 34:163–75.
29. Theofilopoulos AN, Dixon FJ. Autoimmune diseases. Immunopathology and etiopathogenesis. AM J Pathol 1982; 108:321–47.
30. Ziegler JL, Stites DP. Hypothesis: AIDS is an autoimmune disease triggered by a lymphotropic retrovirus. Clin Immunol Immunopathol 1986; 41:305–313.
31. Festenstein H, Awad J, Hitman GA, et al. New DNA polymorphisms associated with autoimmune diseases. Nature 1986; 322:64–7.
32. Taylor JF, Templeton AC, Kyalwazi SK, et al. Kaposi's sarcoma in pregnancy: two case reports. Br J Surg 1971; 58:577–80.
33. Lacey M, Alpert S, Hanakan D. Bovine papilloma virus genome elicits skin tumors in transgenic mice. Nature 1986; 322:609–12.
34. Giraldo G, Beth E. The involvement of cytomegalovirus in acquired immune deficiency syndrome and Kaposi's sarcoma. Prog Allergy 1986; 37:319–31.
35. Wong-Staal F, Ratner L, Shaw G, et al. Molecular biology of human T lymphotropic retroviruses. Cancer Res 1985; 45:4539–47.
36. Gyorkey F, Sinkovics HG, Melnick JL, Gyorkey P. Retroviruses in Kaposi's sarcoma cells in AIDS (letter). N Engl J Med 1984; 311–1183–4.
37. Levy JA, Ziegler JL. Hypothesis. Acquired immunodeficiency syndrome is an opportunistic infection and Kaposi's sarcoma results from secondary immune stimulation. Lancet 1983; 2:78–81.
38. Hohmann EL, Elde RP, Rysavy JA, Einzig S, Gebhard RL. Innervation of periosteum and bone by sympathetic vasoactive intestinal peptide-containing nerve fibers. Science 1986; 232:868–71.
39. Gutman E. Neurotrophic relations. Annu Rev Physiol 1976; 38: 177–216.
40. Safai B, Miké V, Giraldo G, et al. Association of Kaposi's sarcoma with second primary malignancies: possible etiopathogenic implications. Cancer 1980; 45:1472–9.
41. Dollinger MR, Foye LV. Kaposi's sarcoma and coexistent giant follicular lymphoblastoma. Yale J Biol Med 1966; 38:449–55.
42. Ziegler JL, Beckstead JA, Volberding PA, et al. Non-Hodgkin's lymphoma in 90 homosexual men. N Engl J Med 1984; 311:874–9
43. Master SP, Taylor JF, Kyalwazi SK, Ziegler JL. Immunological studies in Kaposi's sarcoma. Br Med J 1970; 1:600–3.
44. Taylor JF, Ziegler JL. Delayed cutaneous hypersensitivity reactions in patients with Kaposi's sarcoma. Br J Cancer 1974; 30:312–8.

45. Bhana D, Templeton AC, Master SP, et al. Kaposi's sarcoma of lymph nodes. Br J Cancer 1970; 24:464–9.
46. Bos JD, Kapsenberg ML. The skin immune system. Its cellular constituents and their interactions. Immunol Today 1986; 7:235–9.
47. Pober JS, Collins T, Gimbrone MA, et al. Lymphocytes recognize human vascular endothelial and dermal fibroblast Ia antigens induced by recombinant interferon. Nature 1983; 305:726–9.
48. Ryan US, Ryan JW, Whitaker L, Chiu A. Fc and C3b receptors on pulmonary endothelial cells: induction by injury. Science 1981; 214:557–9.
49. Warner TFCS, O'Loughlin S. Kaposi's sarcoma. A byproduct of tumor rejection. Lancet 1975; 2:687–9.
50. Birkeland SA, Kemp E, Hauge M. Cancer as a late onset of kidney transplantation. Sci J Urol Nephrol 1977; 42 (Suppl):179–83.
51. Bast RL. Principles of cancer biology: tumor immunotherapy. In: DeVita VT, Hellman S, Rosenberg SA, eds. Cancer. Principles and Practice of Oncology. 2d ed. New York, JB Lippincott, 1985:125–41.
52. Tanaka K, Isselbacher KJ, Khoury G, Jay G. Reversal of oncogenesis by the expression of a major histocompatibility complex class I gene. Science 1985; 228:26–30.
53. McCarthy WD, Pack GT. Malignant blood vessel tumors. A report of 56 cases of angiosarcoma and Kaposi's sarcoma. Surg Gynecol Obstet 1950; 51:465–82.
54. Hiatt HH, Watson JD, Winsten JA. Origin of Human Cancer. Cold Spring Harbor, New York, Cold Spring Harbor Laboratory, 1977: 119–46.
55. Pitot HC. Principles of cancer biology: chemical carcinogenesis. In: DeVita VT, Rosenberg SA, Hellman S, eds. Cancer. Principles and Practice of Oncology. 2d ed. New York, JB Lippincott, 1985:79–97.
56. Sato N, Sato T, Takahashi S, Kikuchi K. Establishment of murine endothelial cell lines that develop angiosarcomas in vivo: brief demonstration of a proposed animal model for Kaposi's sarcoma. Cancer Res 1986; 46:362–6.
57. Ziche M, Gullino PM. Angiogenesis and prediction of sarcoma formation by plastic. Cancer Res 1981; 41:5060–3.
58. Andervont HB, Dunn TB. Effect of castration and sex hormones on the induction of tumors in mice with o-aminoazotoluene. JNCI 1947; 7:455–61.
59. Marmor M, Friedman-Kien AE, Laubenstein L, et al. Risk factors for Kaposi's sarcoma in homosexual men. Lancet 1982; 1:1083–7.

60. Mathur-Wagh U, Mildvan D, Senie RT. Followup at $4\frac{1}{2}$ years on homosexual men with generalized lymphodenopathy (letter). N Engl J Med 1985; 313:1542–3.
61. Haverkos HW, Pinsky PF, Drotman DP, Bergmann DJ. Disease manifestations among heterosexual men with acquired immunodeficiency syndrome (AIDS): a possible role of nitrites in Kaposi's sarcoma. Sex Transm Dis 1985; 12:203–8.
62. Forman D, Al-Dabbagh S, Doll R. Nitrates, nitrites and gastric cancer in Great Britain. Nature 1985; 313:620–5.
63. Goedert JJ, Neuland CY, Wallen WC, et al. Amyl nitrite may alter T lymphocytes in homosexual men. Lancet 1982; 1:412–6.
64. Taylor JF, Iversen OH, Bjerknes R. Growth kinetics of Kaposi's sarcoma. Br J Cancer 1977: 35:470–8.
65. Krigel RK, Friedman-Kien AE. Kaposi's sarcoma in AIDS. In: DeVita VT, Hellman S, Rosenberg SA. AIDS. Etiology, Diagnosis, Treatment, and Prevention. Philadelphia, JB Lippincott, 1985:187–211.
66. Sato N, Goto T, Haranaka K, et al. Actions of tumor necrosis factor on cultured vascular endothelial cells: morphologic modulation, growth inhibition, and cytoxicity. JNCI 1986; 76:1113–21.
67. Bhana D, Hillier K, Karim SMN. Vasoactive substances in Kaposi's sarcoma. Cancer 1971; 27:233–7.
68. Ryan US. Metabolic activity of pulmonary endothelium: modulations of structure and function. Annu Rev Physiol 1986; 48:263–77.
69. Simionescu M, Simionescu N. Functions of the endothelial cell surface. Annu Rev Physiol 1986; 48:279–93.
70. Schnipper LE. Clinical implications of tumor-cell heterogeneity. N Engl J Med 1986; 314:1423–31.
71. Bishop JM. Cancer genes come of age. Cell 1983; 32:1018–20.
72. Weinberg RA. The action of oncogenes in the cytoplasm and nucleus. Science 1985; 230:770–6.
73. Lo SC, Liotta LA. Vascular tumors produced by NIH/3T3 cells transfected with human AIDS Kaposi's sarcoma DNA. Am J Pathol 1985; 118:7–13.
74. Delli Bovi P, Donti E, Knowles DM, et al. Presence of chromosomal abnormalities and lack of AIDS retrovirus DNA sequences in AIDS-associated Kaposi's sarcoma. Cancer Res 1986; 46:6333–8.

2

Pathology

Alexander C. Templeton
Rush Medical College
Presbyterian–St. Luke's Medical Center
Chicago, Illinois

One of the significant impediments to an understanding of this disease is the nomenclature. First, there seems to be no unanimity of opinion about how to pronounce the name of its describer, though the spelling is universally agreed upon. Thus it is much easier to write than to speak about Kaposi's sarcoma. Second, the word *sarcoma* was originally used in a context that did not have the lethal overtones it does now. Today, sarcoma conjures up an image of a quickly growing, locally invasive, destructive, widely metastatic, and rapidly fatal tumor. The sarcoma of Kaposi, however, most often more closely resembles granulation tissue both clinically and histologically, arises in a multicentric fashion, seldom destroys local structures, virtually never metastasizes, and only infrequently disables its host (1).

An accurate diagnosis of whether Kaposi's sarcoma is present in a given individual has very substantial implications for the psychological and physical management of the patient. It is therefore fortunate that in most cases the diagnosis of Kaposi's sarcoma is clinically and histologically obvious. The multiple subcutaneous plaques and/or nodules with their characteristic violaceous hue are almost instantaneously recognizable clinically. Similarly, the histology of the fully formed nodular lesion presents virtually no diagnostic problem. The interlacing of spindle cells and vascular spaces, together with erythrophagocytosis and iron-containing macrophages, is characteristic. These remarks apply to perhaps 80% of cases overall.

The balance of 20% is fraught with problems. These lie in two general areas. First, a locally aggressive tumor mass closely resembles other soft tissue tumors. Second, the distinction of the early lesion of Kaposi's sarcoma from granulation tissue may be difficult. The acquired immunodeficiency syndrome (AIDS) epidemic has increased the diagnostic problems of the histopathologist. Biopsies are now taken from skin lesions that may not yet express the typical histologic appearance of the classic disease. Endoscopic biopsy results in small amounts of tissue for interpretaion. Lymph nodes in AIDS show many changes in addition to Kaposi's sarcoma, which may obscure the histologic picture.

This chapter is not intended to be a comprehensive treatise on the subject of the pathology of this disease, and virtually no material is cited prior to Bluefarb's monograph, published in 1957 (2), to which the reader is referred for the classic references. Another review published in 1976 outlines the African and European disease seen to that point (3). This chapter is concerned predominantly with three aspects of this disease:

1. A recapitulation of the classic disease
2. The diagnosis in the early phase and its distinction from other vascular proliferations
3. The pattern of involvement of different organs, particularly related to the development of symptoms

CLASSIC HISTOPATHOLOGY

The histologic hallmark of Kaposi's sarcoma is a nodule composed of an admixture of spindle cells and small vascular spaces (Figure 1), which appear to arise from a preceding plaque composed mainly of variably shaped blood vessels. In some nodules spindle cells predominate, and in others there are numerous dilated vascular channels resembling a cavernous angioma (Figure 2). The spindle cells are relatively short, regular, and arranged in sheaves. The nuclei are regular with relatively pale chromatin and inconspicuous nucleoli. The nuclear membrane is thin and shows no folds or indentations. The shape is rather more rounded than that seen in smooth muscle or fibroblasts. The cytoplasm is relatively poorly staining, the cell borders are difficult to define, and giant cell formation does not occur. The mitotic rate is usually low, although sometimes a group of cells may show a locally high proportion of mitoses. Red cells are often noted in the interstices between these cells. Sometimes erythrophagocytosis by the spindle cells is noted, a feature that, in this context, is virtually diagnostic of Kaposi's sarcoma. Admixed with these spindle cells are elongated cells

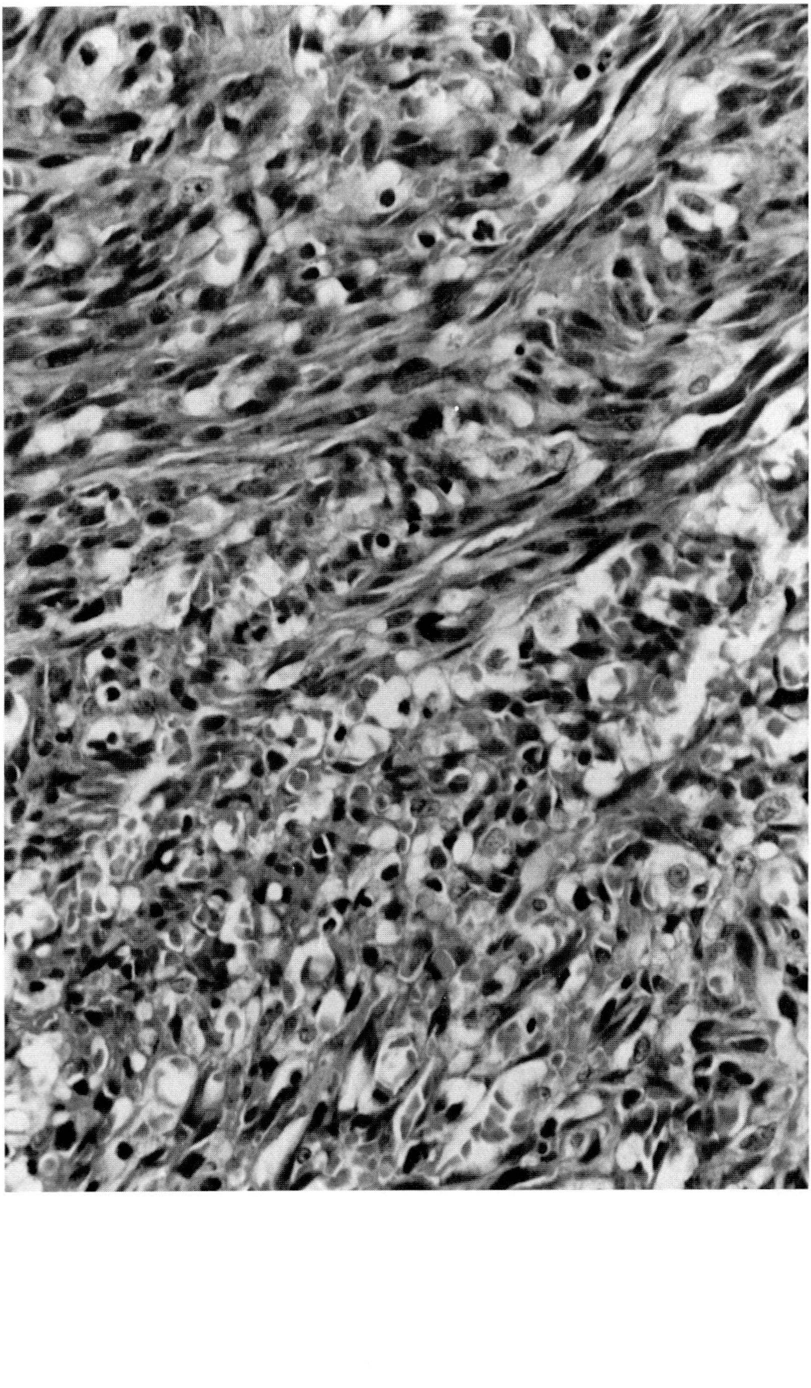

Figure 1 Kaposi's sarcoma, the classic pattern, showing an even mixture of spindle cells and capillary vascular spaces.

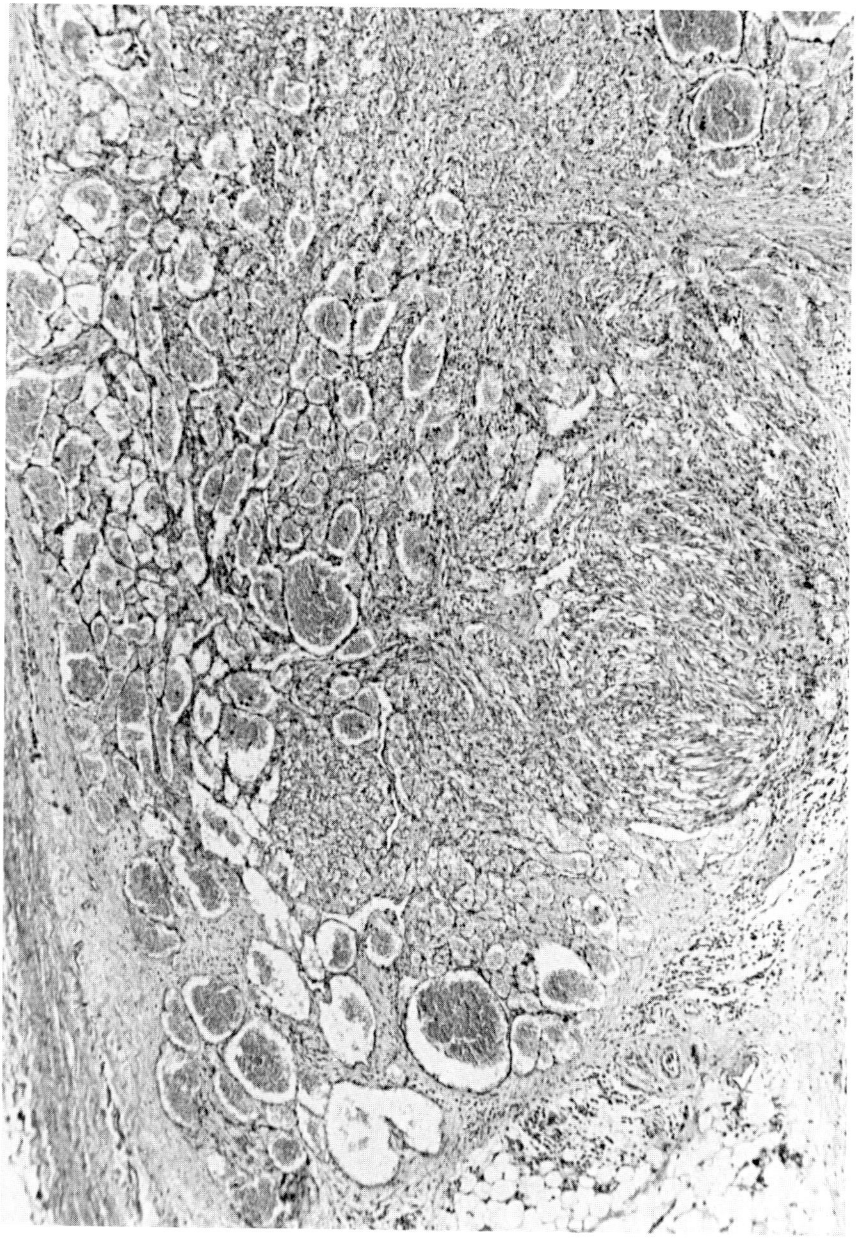

Figure 2 Nodule of Kaposi's sarcoma showing a mixture of classic tumor with dilated spaces resembling cavernous hemangioma.

arranged around lumina, which are formed from only one or two cells with a wall that is only one cell thick. These structures have been referred to as capillary slits and often contain red cells. The lining cells quite frequently show erythrophagocytosis and may contain eosinophilic inclusions (Figure 3). Mitoses are much less commonly seen in this configuration. The nuclei of these two cell types are similar, and it is possible that these are distinct morphological variants of the same cell. The nature of these cells is disputed; this issue is addressed in Chapter 3.

Accompanying this mixture of cells is a proliferation of readily identifiable blood vessels lined by endothelial cells with nuclei that are similar to vessels elsewhere and appear smaller than those in the spindle cells just described. They have defined walls that are distinct and multilayered but often merge into the surrounding tumor. Factor VIII-related antigen can readily be identified in the endothelial cells of these vessels, but there is some controversy about whether this product is present in other cells or merely leached from them to contaminate their neighbors. In most nodules these blood vessels comprise only a small proportion of the tumor and the lumina are small. In some cases throughout the nodule and in others arround the margin, more cavernous vessels are noted with relatively thin walls, again surrounded by a mantle of spindle cells. The lumina may be round as in cavernous hemangiomas of the liver, but more frequently are irregular, elongated, and sometimes apparently branched. These may so dominate the picture that distinction from cavernous hemangioma, lymphangioma, or granuloma pyogenicum becomes difficult (3). The distinction requires the identification of the spindle cells and small luminal spaces already mentioned. It is in this context that the presence of eosinophilic inclusions, resembling morula bodies, is so helpful. Electron microscopy shows these to be lysosomal residual bodies that may be the end result of erythrophagocytosis. The ratio between spindle cells and vascular spaces varies somewhat depending on the clinical context; thus rapidly progressing nodules tend to show a dominance of vascular spaces, whereas nodules that are regressing either

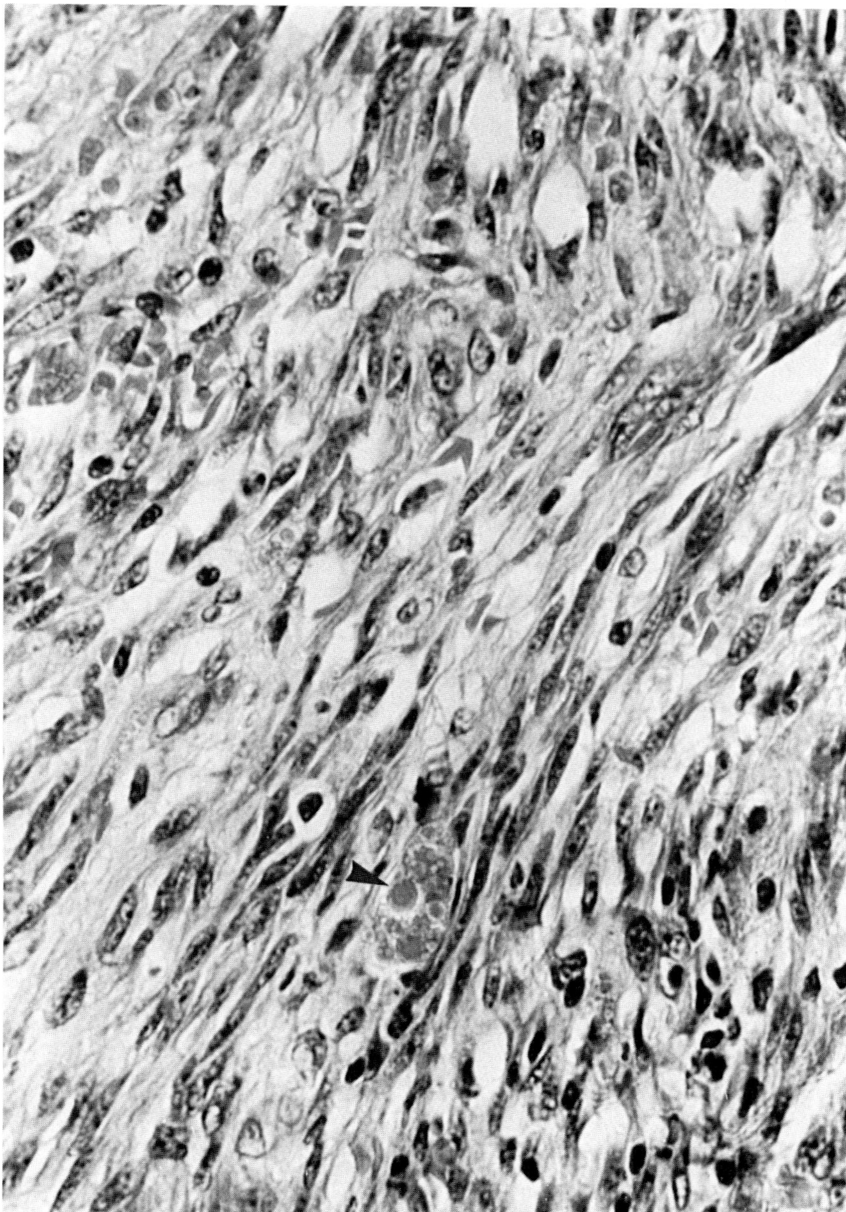

Figure 3 Classic Kaposi's sarcoma; eosinophilic inclusion bodies are noted at the arrow.

spontaneously or under treatment usually show a spindle cell predominance.

The edges of the nodule are usually quite sharp but not entirely encapsulated. In the skin there is almost always a band of relatively normal collagen between the nodule and the epidermis, although this region may contain a few inflammatory cells. A few lymphocytes are usually present at the lateral margins, and these may also be present within the nodule. Plasma cells are usually found but are rarely the predominant cell, except in locally aggressive lesions and nodules within the upper gastrointestinal tract. These inflammatory cells seldom dominate the picture, except when a nodule is clinically regressing and they may then form a prominent collar. In this peripheral zone it is usual to see dilated thin-walled, often misshapen vascular spaces that resemble those seen in the early lesion (see below) and provide evidence that the classic nodule does indeed arise from the vascular plaque stage. The nodule per se rarely penetrates into subcutaneous fat and is never present deep to the deep fascia. Neighboring skin accessories are usually pushed aside but may be incorporated into the nodule, thereby suggesting that little tissue destruction is occurring. The elastica of the surrounding dermis is often fragmented, and the collagen fibers are separated by small pledgelets of tumor insinuating between them. Most nodules of tumor do not ulcerate unless previously traumatized.

Between nodules the skin is often edematous, and dilated vessels, both lymphatic and blood, are commonly observed. In addition, small areas of a vascular proliferation, with some dilated malformed vessels, are seen. This region closely resembles the plaque phase of development and is discussed in more detail below. This proliferation may be present throughout the limb even though the skin appears normal to clinical examination.

The basic histologic pattern is remarkably faithful from region to region and case to case. Thus nodules occurring in the skin, lymph nodes, respiratory tract, and intestines are essentially identical. Similarly, the microscopic picture is the same in virtually all the diverse clinical patterns that may be produced by this tumor.

CLINICAL SUBTYPES

Kaposi himself recognized many of the clinical variants of this disease, but these were not formally codified until 1971, when Kaposi's sarcoma, as seen in Africa, was classified into three major types, some being further divisible (4):

1. Nodular disease
2. Locally aggressive disease
    a. Exophytic
    b. Infiltrative
3. Generalized
    a. Lymphadenopathic
    b. Systemic with or without nodal involvement

Nodular disease encompassed most cases described in the period prior to the mid-1970s. These patients are typically elderly men, usually of African or Southern European ancestry, with subcutaneous acral nodules that grow steadily, often spontaneously resolve, are responsive to treatment by low-dose chemotherapy or radiation therapy, and seldom shorten the life span of the host (Figure 4). Histologically, one notes a diffuse involvement of the dermis of the affected limb. Macroscopically obvious nodules dominate the picture, but in addition the limb is often edematous. The epidermis is usually intact, although it may be somewhat stretched over the surface of the nodule and have a shiny appearance. It is usually discolored and displays a violaceous hue with brownish overtones, so typical of the disease. The skin is not movable over the nodule, but since it only rarely impinges on the subcutaneous fat the nodule is freely mobile on deeper structures. These patients seldom die as a direct result of their disease but usually of unrelated causes. Autopsy studies disclose that many have active systemic nodules or scars suggestive of previous disease, most notably in the gastrointestinal tract (3). Such patients virtually never develop symptoms from this involvement beyond a mild iron-deficiency anemia. Rarely a solitary nodule is noted, and most such patients are apparently cured by excision. Such nodules have been noted on the eyelid, ear, trunk, penis, vulva, and lymph node, among other locations (3). Spontaneous remission of at least a few nodules is noted at some time by virtually every patient with long-standing nodular disease. Histologically this appears to follow one of three distinct pathways. Autoamputation of superficial nodules in the sequence suggested in Figure 5 is common. Another common pattern is the development of a prominent perilesional lymphocytic infiltrate followed by fibrosis and gradual sclerosis of the nodule. The most unusual pattern shows a hemorrhagic expansion of the nodules followed by sclerosis and disappearance of the tumor. On very rare occasions this latter pattern occurs simultaneously in all

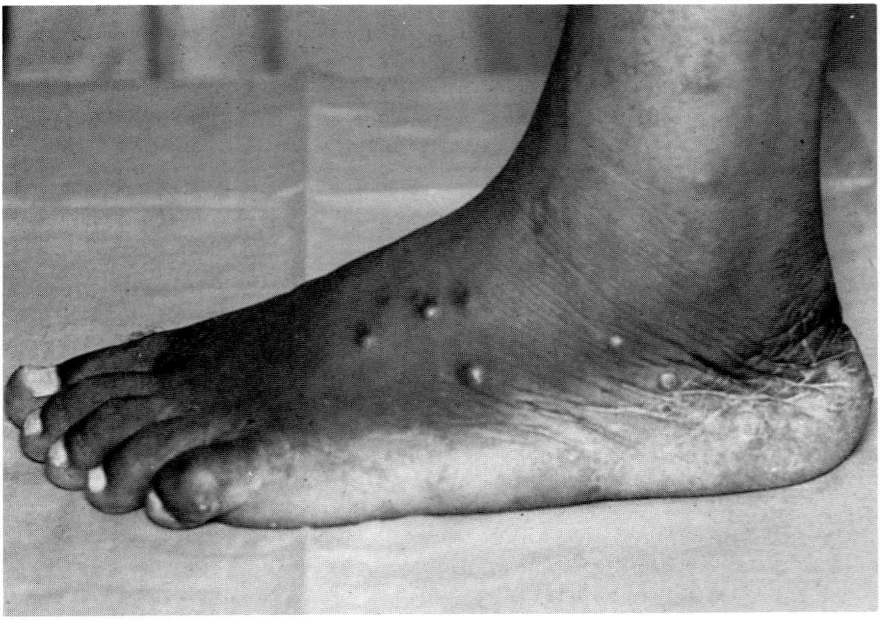

Figure 4 The foot of an African patient with typical nodular disease.

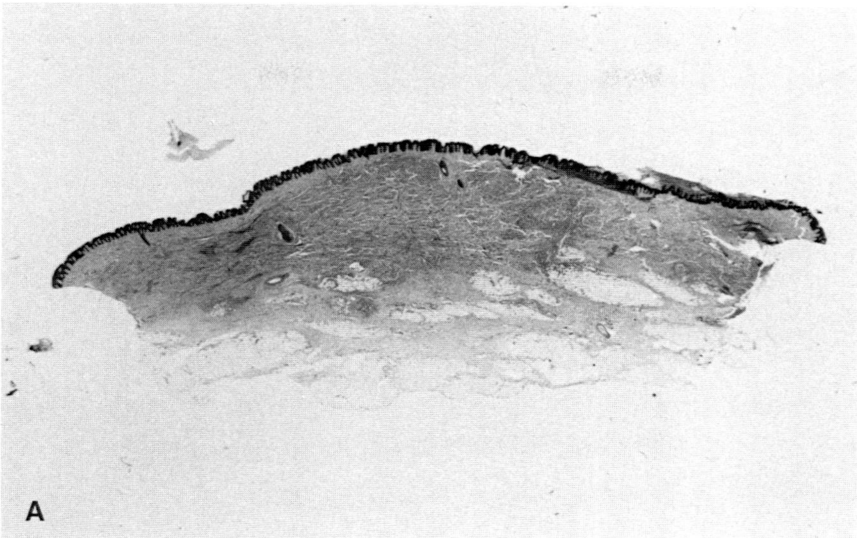

Figure 5 A sequence of cutananeous nodules to show the sequence of events in autoamputation. (A) Plaque-phase disease with wisps of tumor tissue are barely discernible at this power. (B) A Typical nodule; note the relationship to epidermis and deep margins. (C) A nodule of tumor with a well-developed collarette. (D) A tumor nodule that is now pedunculated and ulcerated, with a superimposed pyogenic granuloma-like proliferation.

nodules present, a process strongly reminiscent of hyperacute (thrombotic) rejection of a graft.

Locally aggressive disease usually manifests with an exophytic lesion that both ulcerates and penetrates the deep fascia (Figure 6). In most cases the histologic appearance is identical to that seen within an expansile nodule. Inflammatory infiltration is seldom prominent, but when it occurs it is predominantly of plasma cells. One would have assumed that these clinically sharply different patterns would have been mirrored in their microscopic appearance. Arguing from general neoplastic microscopic principle,

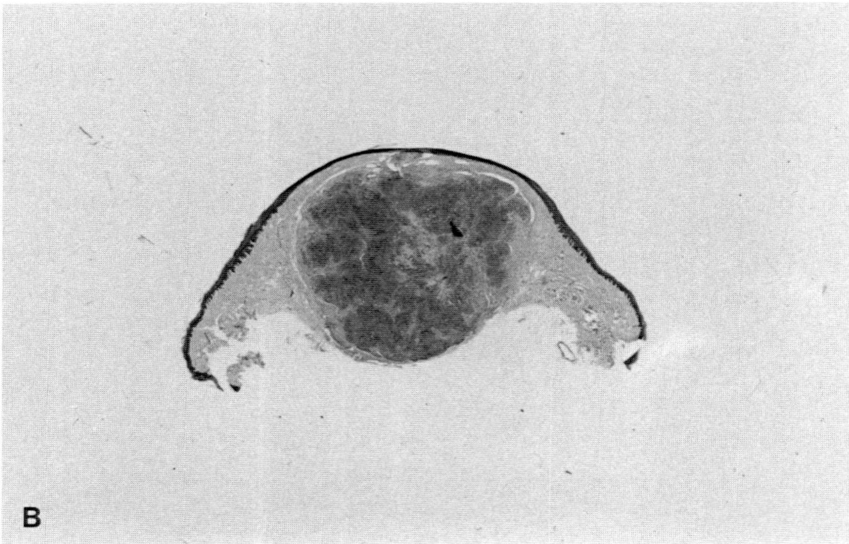

Figure 5B

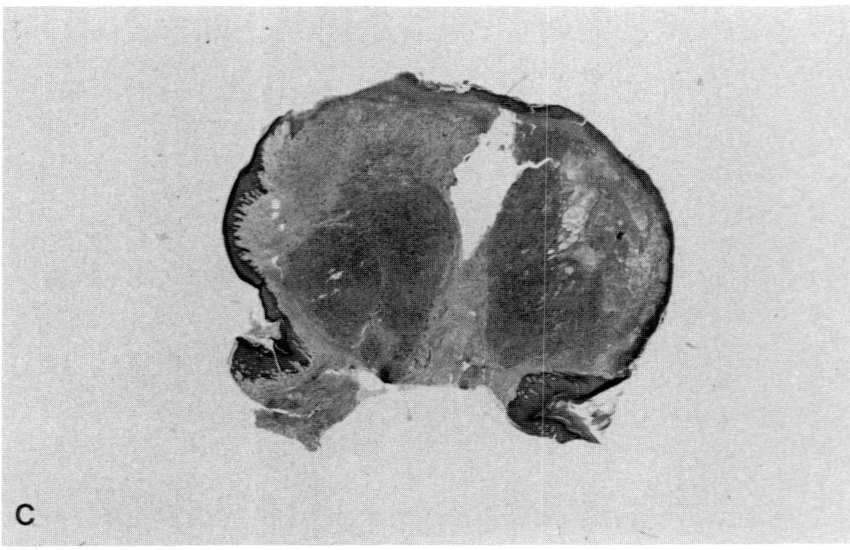

Figure 5C

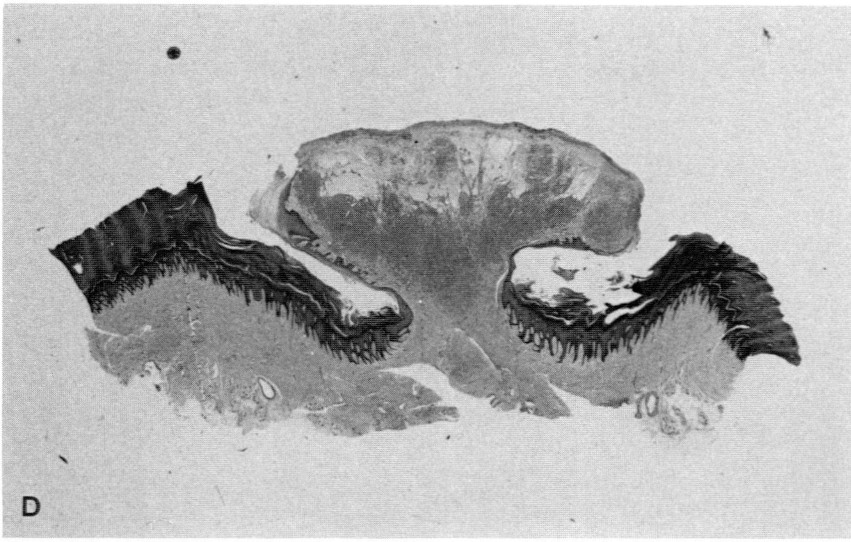

Figure 5D

one might have predicted that larger cells, a higher nuclear-cytoplasmic ratio, more frequent mitoses, or a dominance of spindle cells would be seen in invading tumors. In fact, 60% show an appearance that is identical to that seen in nodular or generalized disease. In the remaining 40% it is difficult to distinguish the histopathologic features from other soft tissue sarcomas, such as hemangiosarcoma or fibrosarcoma. This pattern of disease seems to develop in people who have had nodular disease for some time and may result from further mutations within the genome of tumor cells. However, it is intriguing to note that patients with aggressive disease usually show no response to cutaneous dinitrochlorobenzene (DNCB) challenge, whereas those with nodular disease mount a brisk response. Whether aggressive disease suppresses cutaneous T-cell response or whether immunosuppression allows progression of the disease is uncertain at present.

A less common manifestation of locally aggressive disease is a

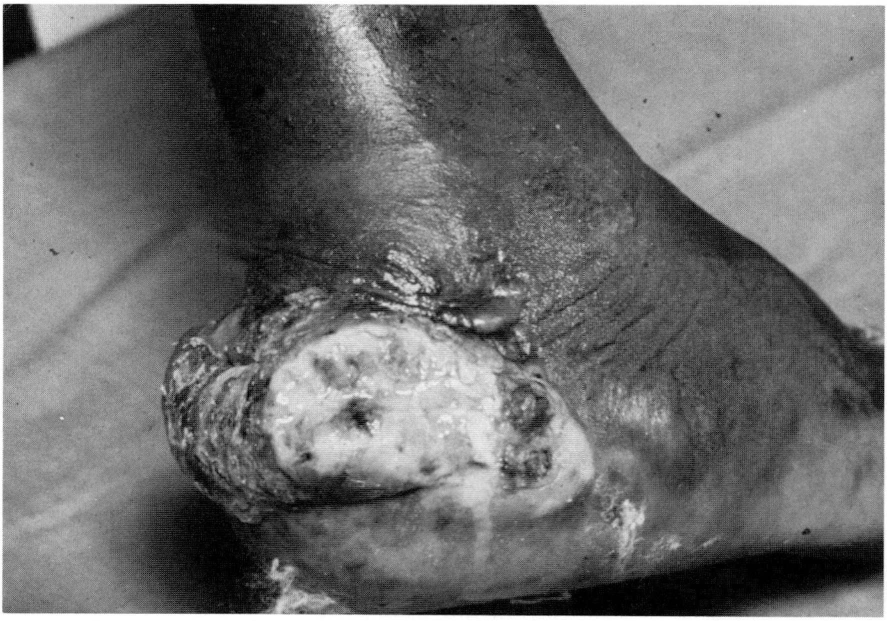

Figure 6 Heel of an African patient with a locally aggressive exophytic tumor mass.

diffusely infiltrative pattern (Figure 7). In such patients the whole limb may become swollen and woody hard.

Generalized disease, either in its lymphadenopathic childhood form or in the systemic disease of young adults, is always characterized by the classic microscopic appearance. Prior to 1980 generalized disease accounted for about 3% of cases in different parts of the world, about half of which occurred in children (5). It has been frequently stated that this pattern was particularly frequent in Africa, but this is not the case. All patterns of disease are more common in Africa than elsewhere, but the generalized form only accounted for the same small proportion as in European subjects, until recently. This form of the disease is characterized by the widespread simultaneous involvement of many different parts of

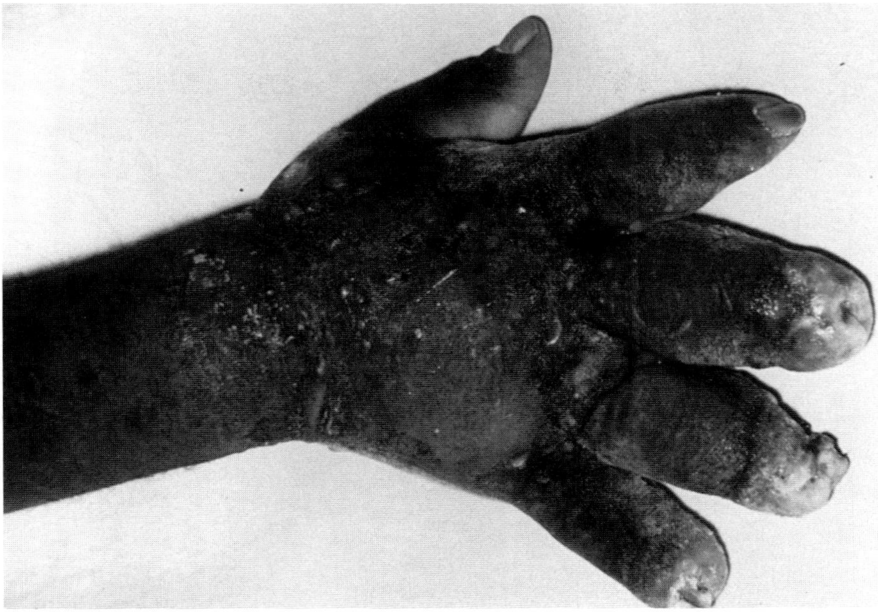

Figure 7 The hand of an African patient with locally aggressive infiltrative disease.

the body with small nodules or plaques. The progress of the disease is rapid, and such patients die within a few weeks unless treatment is instituted. All adults with generalized disease show involvement in many systemic organs, as well as subcutaneous and oral nodules. The gastrointestinal tract, lung, and lymph nodes are most commonly involved. The cause of death in such people is sometimes due to the tumor itself by means of hemorrhage, bronchial obstruction, or intussusception, but in most cases death is a result of generalized inanition. In African patients prior to 1980, *Pneumocystis carinii* infection, disseminated cytomegalovirus infection, or generalized strongyloidiasis was not diagnosed. Children with generalized disease usually have tumor tissue confined to lymph nodes (Figure 8). Girls are affected as often as boys. The cause of

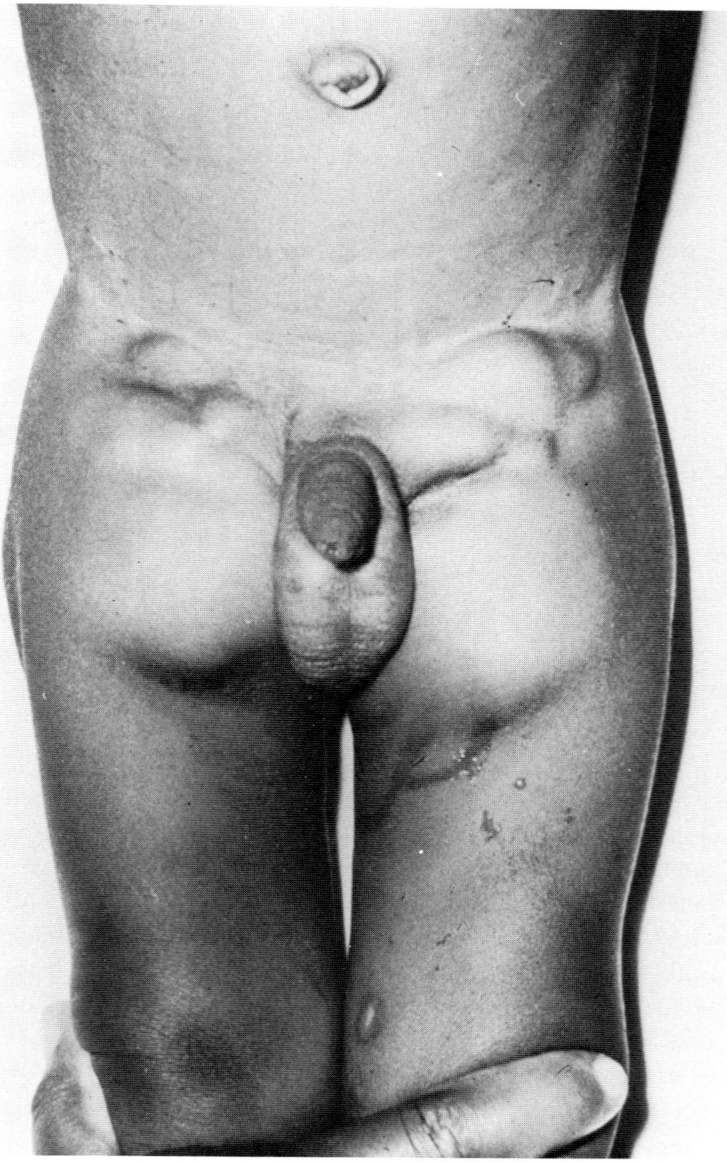

Figure 8 An African child with generalized lymph node enlargement. In spite of their size, the nodes remain remarkably discrete.

death in these children is similarly uncertain; however, it did not appear to be a result of *Pneumocystis* or cytomegalovirus infection. All subjects with this pattern of disease had malaria, and recrudescence of parasitemia contributed to death in many cases.

Prior to the late 1970s, most citizens of Western nations who developed Kaposi's sarcoma exhibited the nodular disease. Scattered reports of childhood lymphadenopathic disease are noted (5), and very few adults with systemic disease were reported (6–10). It is of note that two of these patients were Europeans who were residents for varying periods of time in Africa.

Superimposed upon this distribution are two groups of patients who have been noted to develop Kaposi's sarcoma in recent years. Renal transplant recipients with Kaposi's sarcoma (Chapter 5) usually show nodular disease but may have generalized involvement. Patients with Kaposi's sarcoma developing in association with AIDS show quite a diverse clinical picture. They usually display a generalized pattern of disease that progresses quite rapidly, with simultaneous development of nodules in many areas of the skin, mouth, and systemic mucosae, with respiratory and gastrointestinal involvement particularly common. This is true in Europe, Africa, and America (11–14). There do not appear to be significant differences in clinical pattern or histology of the disease in these different locations, although the "at-risk population" is very different, with women commonly affected in Africa.

The distribution of lesions and histologic picture in the patient with AIDS present an appearance identical to that of Africans with generalized disease prior to 1976. This is not to say that the pathogenesis is the same, because other factors, such as frequency of accompanying cytomegolovirus infection or antibody to human immunodeficiency virus (HIV), are different in these two groups of patients. The histologic picture in the classic European, African, and epidemic AIDS-associated Kaposi's sarcoma is the same (15–17). It is unique in tumor histology that such diverse clinical situations as an elderly European man with indolent subcutaneous nodules, a 20-year-old homosexual male from the United States with oral lesions, a middle-aged patient with a rapidly growing destructive metastasizing tumor mass on the leg, and an African child with generalized lymphadenomegaly should all show an identical histologic picture. Personal experience, measuring the size and shape of spindle cells, the size and shape of nuclei and nucleoli, the mitotic index, size and proportion of vascular structures, and inflammatory infiltrate in tumors from different parts of the world have shown that all these parameters are the same in virtually all cases.

EVOLUTION OF CUTANEOUS KAPOSI'S SARCOMA

The earliest clinical sign of involvement of the skin in all patients developing Kaposi's sarcoma is the development of a cyanotic pink patch. The skin is not raised, and the epidermis appears normal. This phase of the disease is seldom diagnosed except in the context of AIDS. In Africans, skin pigmentation obscures these changes and elderly individuals are not attuned to taking skin blemishes on their feet particularly seriously. Biopsy at this stage shows a proliferation of slightly ectatic vessels, usually grouped around the skin accessories or more superficially placed, with an adjacent mild lymphocytic infiltrate (Figure 9A). The lumina of these vessels usually contain few red cells, and the endothelial cells are no more prominent than in most perivascular diseases. The major differential diagnosis at this point comprises posttraumatic or infectious granulation tissue (18). These latter two lesions are usually associated with reactive epidermal proliferation, and a few polymorphonuclear leucocytes are present in the area. These are conspicuous by their absence in most cases of Kaposi's sarcoma. However, the known propensity of Kaposi's sarcoma to arise in an area of previous trauma does make for a difficult distinction in many cases. With these changes alone Kaposi's sarcoma cannot be diagnosed with certainty.

Within this rather nonspecific pattern more suspicious features then appear. A vascular proliferation is noted, most commonly within the reticular dermis. In a number of cases it may be more superficially placed, but never does it involve the subcutaneous fat. A few of these vessels have a large lumen, a thin wall, and many apparent branches or points from the major lumen. The endothelial nuclei are almost always normal without significant atypia; in fact, they are usually smaller than those seen in a conventional healing wound. These vessels are located between adjacent collagen bundles and separate them one from the other. Extravasation of red cells is almost always found if sought but is seldom prominent. Iron-containing macrophages are a common feature of endemic disease on the foot but are rarely prominent in the epidemic form, particularly from lesions in the upper part of the body. Inflammatory cells are few in number, but in contrast to usual healing granulation tissue there are lymphocytes with a few macrophages and/or plasma cells but no polymorphonuclear leukocytes (Figure 9B). This has been referred to as the patch stage of the lesion (19). Opinion varies about how reliable are diagnoses made on changes at this point. It may be that a subgroup of patients at high risk for developing Kaposi's sarcoma can be delineated by finding such changes, even by biopsy of clinically normal skin (20).

The next diagnostically useful change is the appearance of spindle cells between the vascular spaces. It is at this stage that a firm diagnosis of plaque-phase Kaposi's sarcoma can be made (Figure 9C). Nuclear abnormalities can now be noted in the cells lining vascular spaces. Mitoses may be present, and nuclear variability is more marked than heretofore. However, nucleoli are not prominent and the nuclear membranes do not show the irregular thickening of more conventional malignant cells. The spindle cell nuclei often appear more aggressive in that mitoses are easier to find and nucleoli are prominent, but in only a few cells is hyperchromatism noted. Extravasation of red cells is much easier to detect at this point, and hemosiderin-laden macrophages, although seldom prominent, are almost always present. Eosinophilic inclusions are readily seen in most African cases, particularly in the vascular areas, and in a high proportion of oral lesions (21).

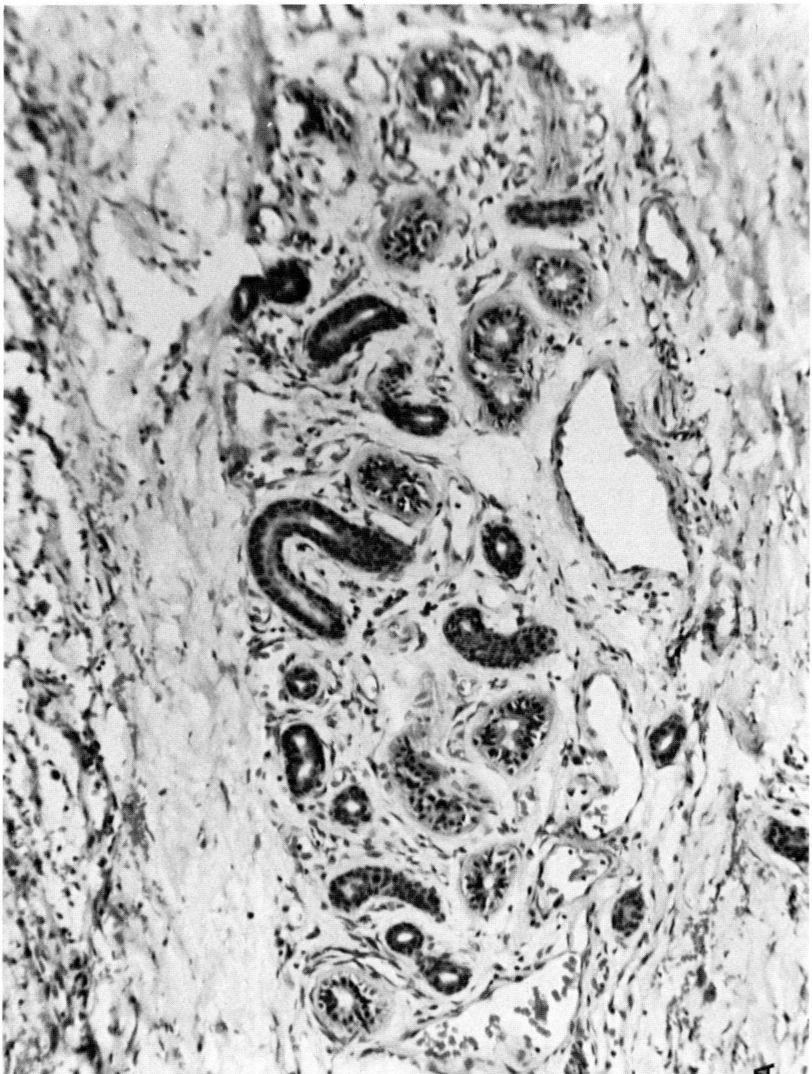

Figure 9 A sequence of views from the same skin biopsy illustrated in Figure 5 showing the development of Kaposi's sarcoma at the level of skin accessary glands. (A) Edema and a few inflammatory cells are present around sweat glands.

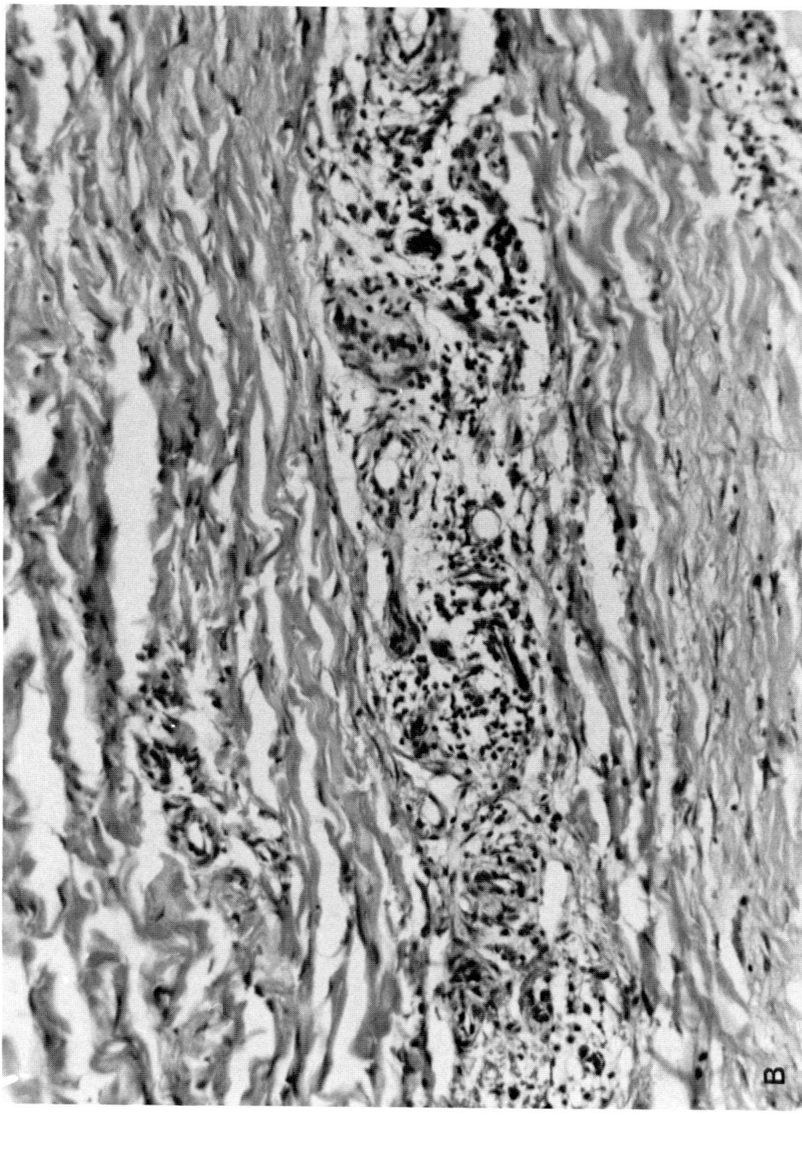

Figure 9B The appearance is now of inflammatory granulation tissue.

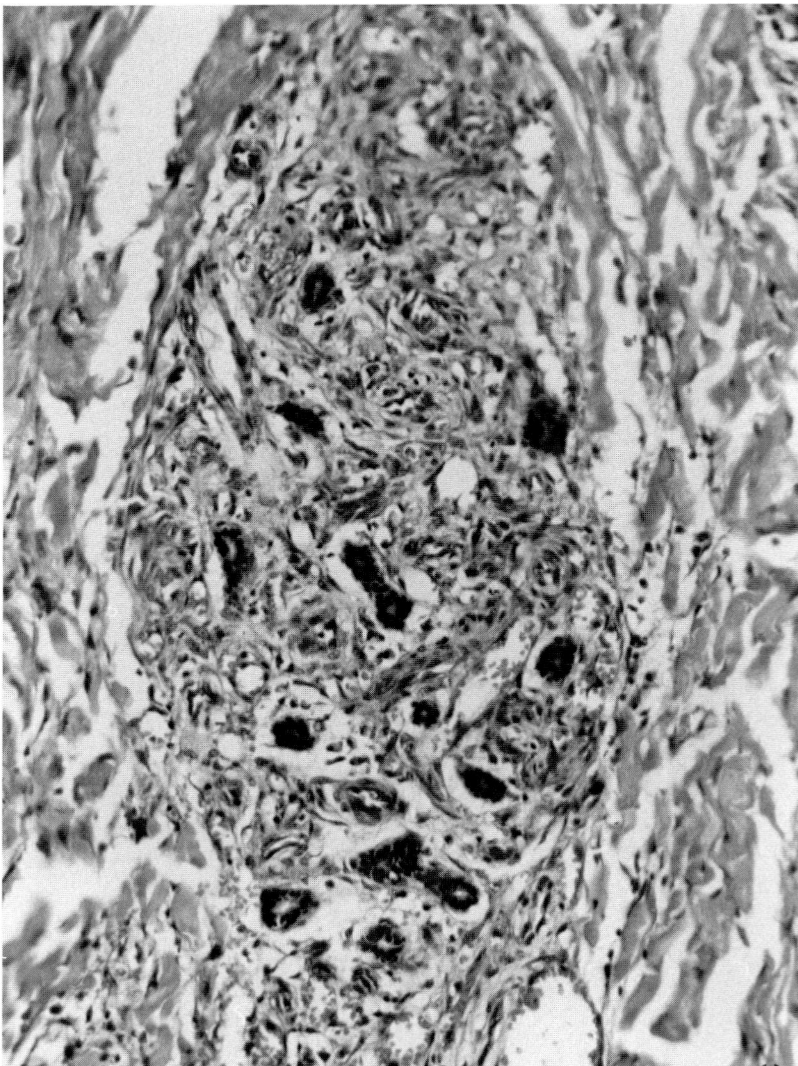

Figure 9C Plaque-phase Kaposi's sarcoma is now diagnosable.

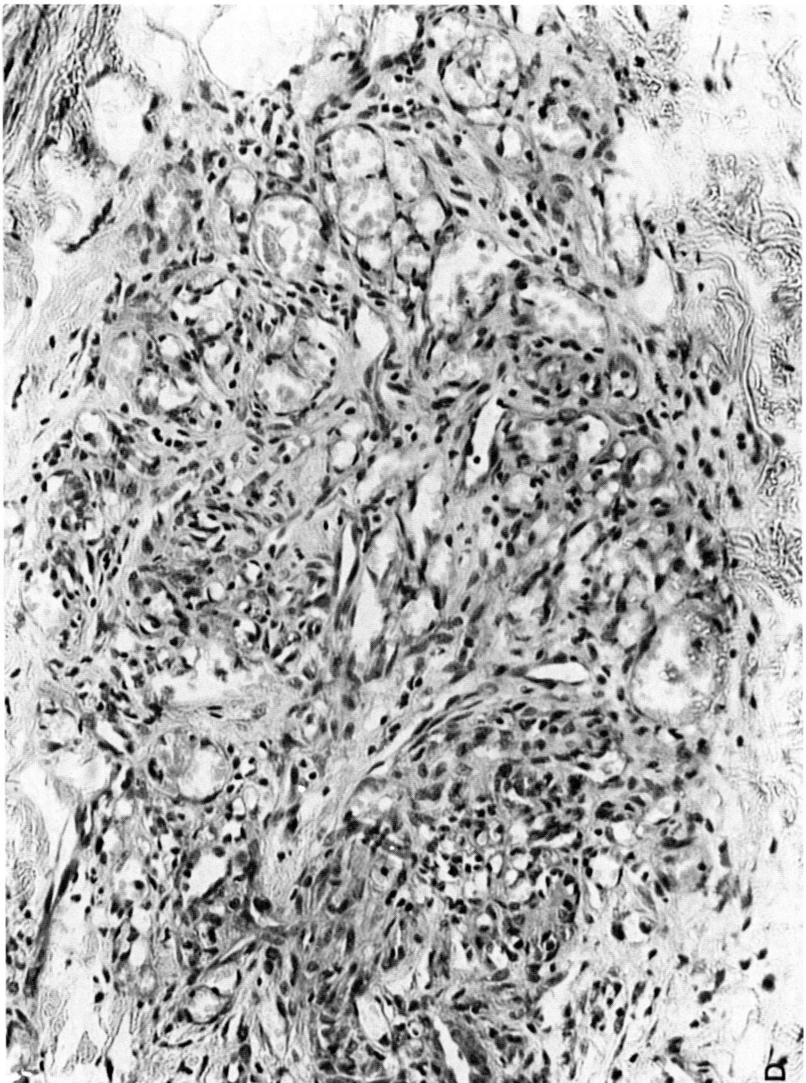

Figure 9D A nodule has now developed, and the skin accessory structures are pushed aside.

Although these are less apparent in most AIDS-related cutaneous lesions they can almost invariably be found if patiently sought.

Within a plaque, proliferation of vascular and spindle cells continues to produce the nodule so typical of the disease in its classic form (Figure 9D). Residua of the plaque stage are usually identifiable at the shoulders of small nodules, although they disappear around larger lesions. Elsewhere in the adjacent skin nonspecific vascular proliferation is usually visible.

DIFFERENTIAL DIAGNOSIS

Clinical

Differential diagnosis is rather different in the three major groups of clinical types of Kaposi's sarcoma. In elderly Europeans, nodular disease is difficult to distinguish from stasis dermatitis, both clinically and histologically (19,20). This problem is addressed below. In Africans with nodular disease the clinical diagnoses considered include leprosy and *Tunga penetrans* infection, among others. Histology, however, is usually distinctive. In patients with locally aggressive lesions, distinction from such infections as maduramycosis and mossy foot may pose problems. Other soft tissue tumors may be next to impossible to distinguish both clinically and histologically. Many locally aggressive lesions show the classic appearance of Kaposi's sarcoma, very similar to that seen in a nodule, and others show a spindle cell preponderance. A few aggressive tumors do not resemble the appearance of Kaposi's sarcoma at all and show the histologic picture of hemangiosarcoma (Figure 10). Diagnosis of Kaposi's sarcoma in such lesions is usually achieved by noting the classic appearance in nodules elsewhere in the same patient. These tumors invade and metastasize widely and do not respond to chemotherapy as do aggressive Kaposi's sarcoma lesions with a more conventional appearance. Perhaps such tumors may be better regarded as distinctly different tumors arising in a patient with Kaposi's sarcoma rather than as a variant of the disease. The

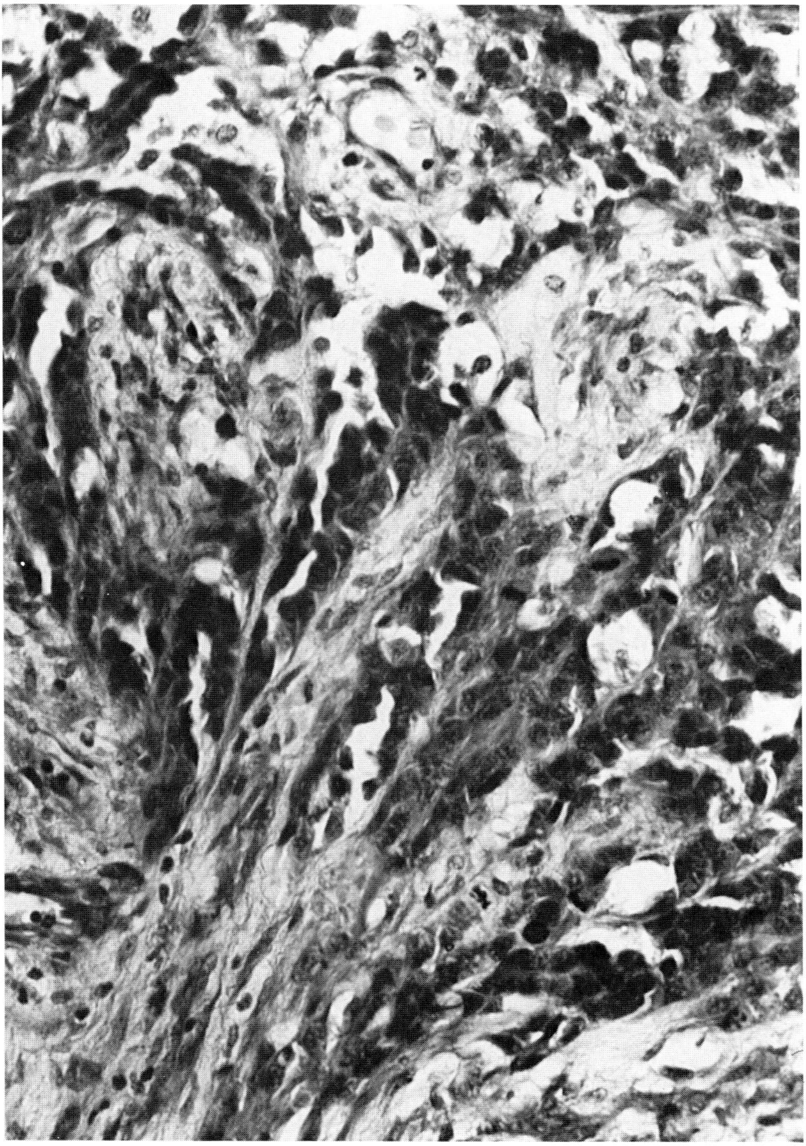

Figure 10 Pleomorphic pattern of tumor resembling hemangiosarcoma. This particular tumor showed typical Kaposi's sarcoma elsewhere in the mass.

generalized lymphadenopathic form of childhood disease is difficult to distinguish from lymphoma clinically, but the diagnosis of Kaposi's sarcoma is obvious histologically. Similarly, generalized disease in adults is sometimes confused for subcutaneous parasitic disorders but is almost always readily identifiable microscopically.

The clinical differential diagnosis of cutaneous lesions in AIDS is wide (22–24) and apart from Kaposi's sarcoma includes infections by *Histoplasma*, *Cryptococcus*, *Candida*, *Mycobacteria*, or *Acanthameba*; nutritional disorders, such as pellagra; and neoplasms, such as malignant lymphoma. A biopsy is usually recommended in such cases, but if plaques of violet shade are noted forming on the trunk, mouth, or proximal limbs, the clinical diagnosis of Kaposi's sarcoma is rarely contradicted by light microscopy.

Histologic Differential Diagnosis: Plaque Phase

The differential diagnosis from stasis dermatitis, although very difficult on a microscope slide, is a problem that is more apparent than real. Patients with AIDS seldom have congestion of their limbs nor do they develop lesions in endematous areas. In an elderly patient with stasis in the limb, if there is doubt about the diagnosis, a biopsy at a later date will usually clarify the issue. Delay is of little consequence in this indolent pattern of disease, which does not require therapy early in its course. Both conditions show a prominent vascular proliferation, extravasation of red cells, iron-containing macrophages, some sclerosis in the surrounding dermis, moderate numbers of inflammatory cells, and a tendency to aggregate in either the deep or superficial plexus of cutaneous vessels. The essence of the distinction is the appearance of three features in lesions of Kaposi's sarcoma. Perivascular spindle cell proliferation is the most important, but in early lesions this may be minimal and difficult to distinguish from perivascular fibrosis seen in chronically congested tissues. Erythrophagocytosis by spindle cells is almost pathognomonic when seen, but to be identified a fair number of spindle cells have to be present and in early lesions this feature is difficult to confirm. It is easier to confirm on electron microscopy than on light microscopy, but the presence of variably sized eosinophilic fragments can usually be identified as portions of red cells on hematoxylin and eosin-stained paraffin sections. The third feature is the development of clustered eosinophilic cytoplasmic inclusions. Electron microscopy is useful in making these distinctions in problem cases since Kaposi's sarcoma vessels show incomplete or absent perithelial investment, discontinuity of the endothelial cells, some necrotic cells, and incomplete basement membrane formation (22). Stasis dermatitis, in contrast, shows a thickening of basement membrane. The capillary sprouts of granulation tissue usually show a readily identifiable perithelial investment, and although the endothelial layer may be incomplete the basement membrane is usually complete.

The distinction of Kaposi's sarcoma from the lymphatic channel proliferation seen in lymphedematous limbs is much more problematic histologically since these also show an incomplete endothelial layer and an absence of perithelial investment. Mercifully this distinction is seldom one that a pathologist has to make since both Milroy's disease and acquired lymphedema of microfilariasis are readily identified clinically and seldom biopsied.

Histologic Differential Diagnosis: Nodular Phase

The group of conditions that may be confused with the nodular phase of Kaposi's sarcoma share a common feature of spindle and vascular proliferation. Dermatofibroma, angiolipoma, histiocytoid hemangioma, spindle cell hemangioendothelioma, acroangiodermatitis, intravascular papillary endothelial hyperplasia, and various posttraumatic proliferations, such as granuloma pyogenicum and scars, have to be recognized and distinguished (25–35). Knowledge of the clinical appearance of the disease and information about multiplicity, presence in a female, and the age and recent history of the patient considerably assist interpretation.

The recently described spindle cell hemangioendothelioma

(25) very closely resembles classic Kaposi's sarcoma in its clinical picture. This lesion may occur at virtually any age and presents as solitary or multiple nodules on the limb. These progress slowly over months or sometimes years and do not metastasize until late in the course of the disease. Prior to this description the presence of multiple lesions developing in an edematous limb would have been regarded by most clinicians as virtually pathognomonic of Kaposi's sarcoma, but on occasion this picture develops with spindle cell hemangioendothelioma. Histologically, the tumor shows a mixture of spindle cells and small vessels that in small areas may mimic Kaposi's sarcoma exactly. Distinction largely depends on the relationship of the tumor to large vessels. Spindle cell hemangioendothelioma usually shows endovascular proliferation, which may precipitate thrombosis in which calcification sometimes occurs. These features are seldom seen in Kaposi's sarcoma. Endovascular proliferation is sometimes seen in locally aggressive tumors but is never prominent. Dilated vessels with thrombosis and phleboliths are distinctly unusual in Kaposi's sarcoma.

Lesions that occur predominantly within the lumen of blood vessels are more easy to distinguish from Kaposi's sarcoma. Masson's vegetant intravascular hemangioendothelioma is probably not a neoplasm but is more likely a reactive condition that represents a peculiar pattern of organization within a venous thrombus (26,27). A similar picture may occur within lymphatic channels (28). This lesion usually occurs as a solitary nodule, and the papillary endovascular nature of the proliferations seen histologically readily distinguishes these lesions from Kaposi's sarcoma. However, rare cases of multiple nodular proliferations occur that make clinical distinction difficult.

The precise nature of acroangiodermatitis (29–31) and its relationship to arteriovenous fistulas are debated. The resemblance of this condition to Kaposi's sarcoma is so close that the term "pseudo-Kaposi's sarcoma" is often used to describe it. Biopsy of an abnormal vascular prolifertion around an acquired arteriovenous fistula is one situation in which electron microscopy is often necessary to make a distinction of reactive from neoplastic disorder. As noted, Kaposi's sarcoma shows no perithelial investment and an incomplete basement membrane, whereas acroangiodermatitis usually shows marked thickening of the basal laminae with numerous perithelial cells (32).

Fibrohistiocytic lesions are usually easy to distinguish from Kaposi's sarcoma since they are most often solitary and do not contain a vascular component histologically. Multiple dermatofibromas do occur rarely in AIDS patients, as do angiolipomas (33) and these may cause some diagnostic problems clinically. Angiomatoid variants of either benign (34) or malignant (35) fibrous histiocytomas are sometimes confused for Kaposi's sarcoma histologically. Benign angiomatoid (aneurysmal) fibrous histiocytoma also usually presents as a solitary mass on the limb (34). The characteristic story is that of nodule that has been present for years and has recently become painful and enlarged. The histologic distinction is relatively straightforward since the small capillary slits so typical of Kaposi's sarcoma are absent. However organization of a thrombus within angiomatoid fibrous histiocytoma may produce a mixture of components of vascular spaces and spindle cells that may resemble Kaposi's sarcoma in areas. Other regions of the lesion show spindle cell preponderance, and a few giant cells are often present. Malignant angiomatoid fibrous histiocytoma usually occurs in children (one-third of patients are aged 20 or above) and presents as a solitary subcutaneous nodule on the limb. The histopathology shows a much more aggressive appearance than that of the usual Kaposi's nodule. Giant cells are common, and there is often prominent nuclear pleomorphism together with chronic inflammatory infiltrate. The group of conditions known variously as histiocytoid or epithelioid hemangioma are usually sharply distinguishable from Kaposi's sarcoma, although a report concerning a 55-year-old male with abnormal helper-suppressor lymphocyte ratio who had such a lesion with apparent transition to areas resembling Kaposi's sarcoma is of considerable interest (36).

DISTRIBUTION OF LESIONS

It is difficult to obtain reliable statistics about the frequency of involvement of different organs in patients with Kaposi's sarcoma.

This is because different criteria are often used in the denominator and numerator of this ratio. Thus some series diagnose involvement of an organ only in those patients who develop symptoms referable to this location, some are based on patients in whom an active search for tumor has occurred with endoscopy or radiology, and yet others on autopsy data. In addition, the incidence of involvement varies with the clinical type of disease present and this in turn is influenced by the institution from which the report emanates. Even if the reports are restricted to AIDS-related patients in whom autopsy studies have been conducted, there appears to be wide variation in frequency of involvement suggesting variations in both time and place as well as diagnostic criteria (37). When individual organs or sites are considered these variations are more marked; thus nodal involvement is noted in 20–90% (37) and oral involvement in 5–50% (21). This section is therefore confined to description of the pattern of involvement in each site and firm incidence figures, which are likely to be challenged and possibly change radically as the epidemic of Kaposi's sarcoma matures, are avoided.

Cutaneous Lesions

Cutaneous involvement is by far the most common manifestation of Kaposi's sarcoma seen in the clinic and is usually the lesion that leads to diagnosis. In the classic nodular form of the disease acral involvement is the first sign, and fresh nodules appear in a centripetal fashion. Rarely an isolated nodule occurs at an ectopic site, but involvement of the skin of the face or trunk is rather unusual even in long-standing disease. In AIDS-associated patients the distribution is more capricious. The face, trunk, buttocks, and proximal limbs may each or all be involved before acral involvement occurs. Small plaques occur, and these may grow rapidly but rarely exceed a centimeter in diameter. The nodules of AIDS-associated tumors are seldom quite as protuberant as those of the classic type. Classic nodular Kaposi's sarcoma often occurs in association with and appears to accelerate edema of the limb, but this is seldom so in the

AIDS-associated disease. In both situations the tumor appears to arise at the level of the superficial plexus of vessels and rarely causes spontaneous ulceration or penetration deep to the deep fascia. Thus, although many authors use the terms "malignant" and "metastasis" in describing cutaneous Kaposi's sarcoma, this is really not justified in all but the locally aggressive form seen in Africans.

Mouth and Gastrointestinal Tract

The next most common site of clinically diagnosed involvement is the gastrointestinal tract (38–40). Scattered nodules are found in a significant proportion of patients with classic nodular disease, but this is rarely of great clinical significance. AIDS-associated Kaposi's sarcoma frequently shows involvement of the gastrointestinal tract. Oral disease is very commonly seen, particularly when actively sought, and may be the initial sign of disease (2). Plaques are most commonly noted on the palate, but the gingiva, tongue, or buccal mucosa may be involved. Oral lesions are made up of a greater proportion of spindle cells than is usual in the skin and the inflammatory cells present are more likely to be plasma cells, but otherwise histology is very similar to that seen in other parts of the body. In most instances these lesions do not produce obvious nodules, although polypoid masses that may bleed, ulcerate, and become secondarily infected are noted. A majority of patients with oral involvement show lesions elsewhere in the gastrointestinal tract (40). In the pharynx and esophagus a greater proportion of diagnosed lesions are nodular proliferations, and these may become ulcerated or infected and cause hemorrhage or obstruction.

In the stomach the pattern of disease is variable. The whole of the gastric mucosa may be involved in a sheetlike plaque closely mimicking the appearance of acute gastritis, or a variable number of polyps may be noted. Ulceration, which may be identifiable radiologically as an umbilicated nodule or hemorrhage, is very commonly seen in this location and subsequent hemorrhage occurs frequently. Small intestinal nodules are commonly seen at autopsy but are not frequently diagnosed during life. These develop under the submucosa and may become pedunculated, when ulceration (Figure 11), hemorrhage, and intussusception may develop. Colonic involvement is common and most usually exhibits numerous nodules that develop ulceration and hemorrhage. Colonic nodules are usually very dark in color as a result of hemorrhage and infection, whereas nodules higher in the gastrointestinal tract are usually redder. More rarely a diffuse involvement of the bowel is noted, and this may be difficult to distinguish from pseudomembranous colitis or one of the many infectious causes of colitis seen in this population.

At all these sites the evolution and histologic appearance are similar. The lesion appears to develop in the submucosa through the same stages as noted in the skin. The plaque phase gives rise to few symptoms and is seldom biopsied, but such lesions are commonly discovered at autopsy. Involvement of the underlying muscularis propria is rare, and penetration of the serosa or perforation is extremely rare but has been reported once (41). Superficial biopsies taken through endoscopic instruments are often negative since, although intramucosal lesions do occur (40), most nodules are located in the submucosa. Patients with gastrointestinal lesions are reported to have a poorer prognosis (39) and a greater degree of immune suppression (40). The wisdom of attempting biopsy of these lesions may be questioned since complicating hemorrhage may occur, and histologic validation of disease is often not forthcoming since the tumor is usually located deep within the submucosa.

Respiratory Tract

The frequency of involvement of the respiratory tract varies with the clinical type of disease present. A very small proportion of patients with nodular endemic Kaposi's sarcoma may show an isolated pulmonary nodule. In this context, however, such an x-ray appearance is much more likely to be due to accompanying granulomatous disease. Patients with locally aggressive disease may show pulmonary metastasis as with other sarcomas, but this is also

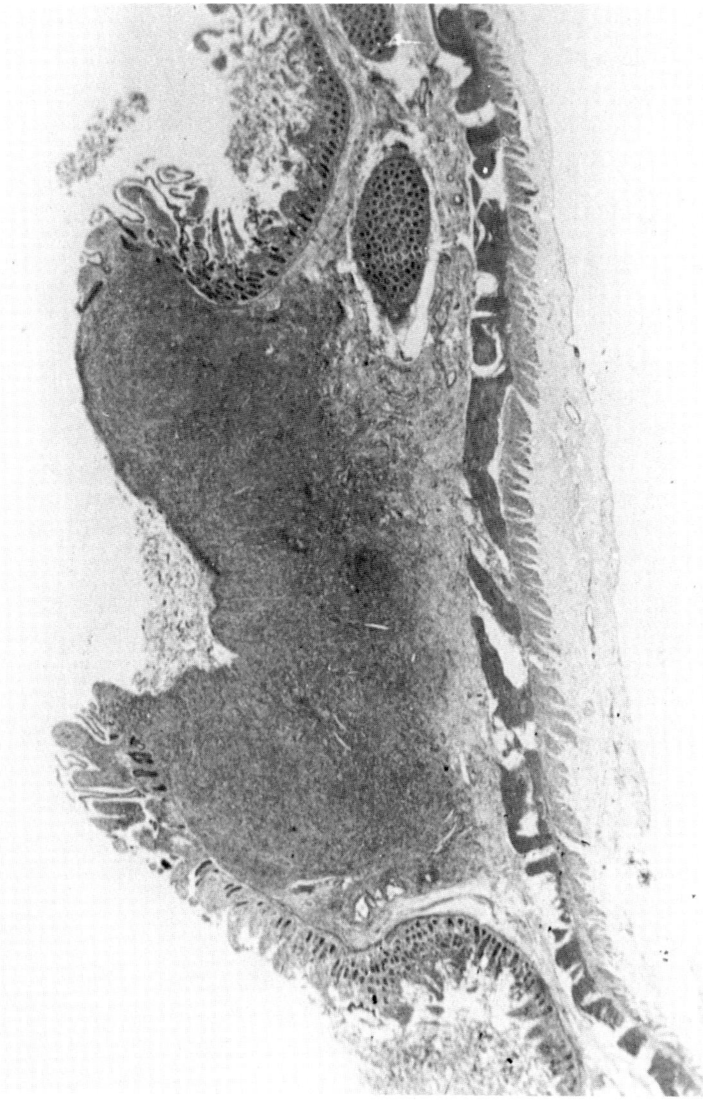

Figure 11 Nodule of Kaposi's sarcoma in the small intestine, showing ulceration and characteristic umbilication.

unusual. Patients with AIDS-associated disease develop pulmonary involvement in about 50% of cases, and the tumor contributes to death in about one-quarter of these cases (42–47). For this reason, identification of pulmonary involvement is an indication for immediate treatment.

Tumor in the respiratory tract shows features very similar to those seen in other parts of the body. Plaques and nodules are both present and comprise an admixture of spindle cells and small vascular lumina with a variable mixture of inflammatory cells. There are some differences, however. First, the tumor most commonly grows as a sheet rather than a nodule, and second, there tends to be a predominance of spindle cells (Figure 12) rather than an equal admixture of spindle and vascular spaces. In the tracheobronchial tree, plaques and nodules may be seen as at other sites. Diagnosis can sometimes be made on plain x-ray when impingement by tumor on the air bronchogram is particularly marked. More usually diagnosis is made by bronchoscopy. The interpretation of biopsies taken at bronchoscopy is usually straightforward. The presence of a vascular and/or pleomorphic spindle cell proliferation under unbroken epithelium is strongly suggestive of Kaposi's sarcoma. When ulceration is present, with the inevitable accompanying granulation tissue, the diagnosis is much more difficult. There is some controversy about whether biopsy of such lesions should be undertaken. Pulmonary involvement may be the first site in which Kaposi's sarcoma is diagnosed (43), but more commonly the diagnosis has been established by cutaneous or oral biopsy. In the latter case the risk of biopsy probably outweighs the potential beneift since tracheobronchial infections can be diagnosed quite efficiently by brush or lavage.

Tracheal tumors may grow large enough to occlude the airway (Figure 13) (46). Parenchymal involvement, in contrast, usually fails to show an identifiable mass. The tumor grows as a sheath around bronchi, pulmonary vessels (Figure 14), pulmonary septae, and under the pleura. At all these sites it appears to follow quite faithfully the distribution of pulmonary lymphatics. Clinical and radiologic distinction from viral pneumonia is very difficult, and

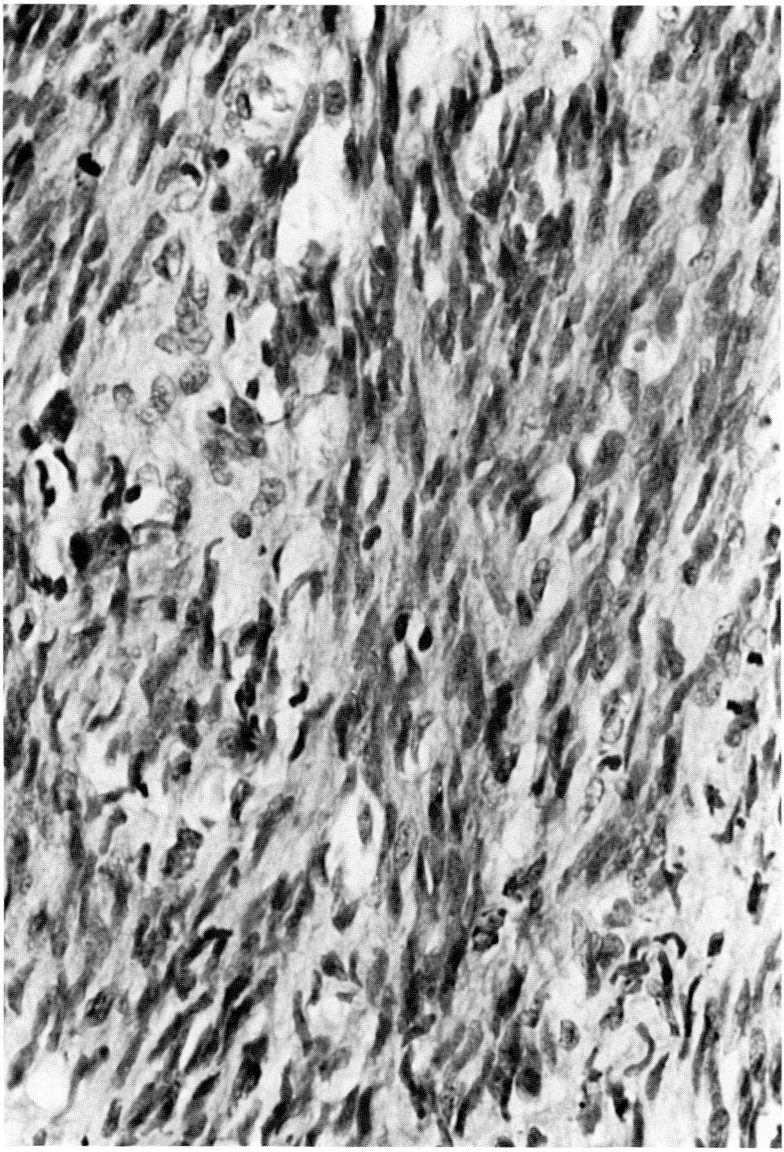

Figure 12 Photomicrograph showing the spindle cell preponderance often found in Kaposi's sarcoma within the lung.

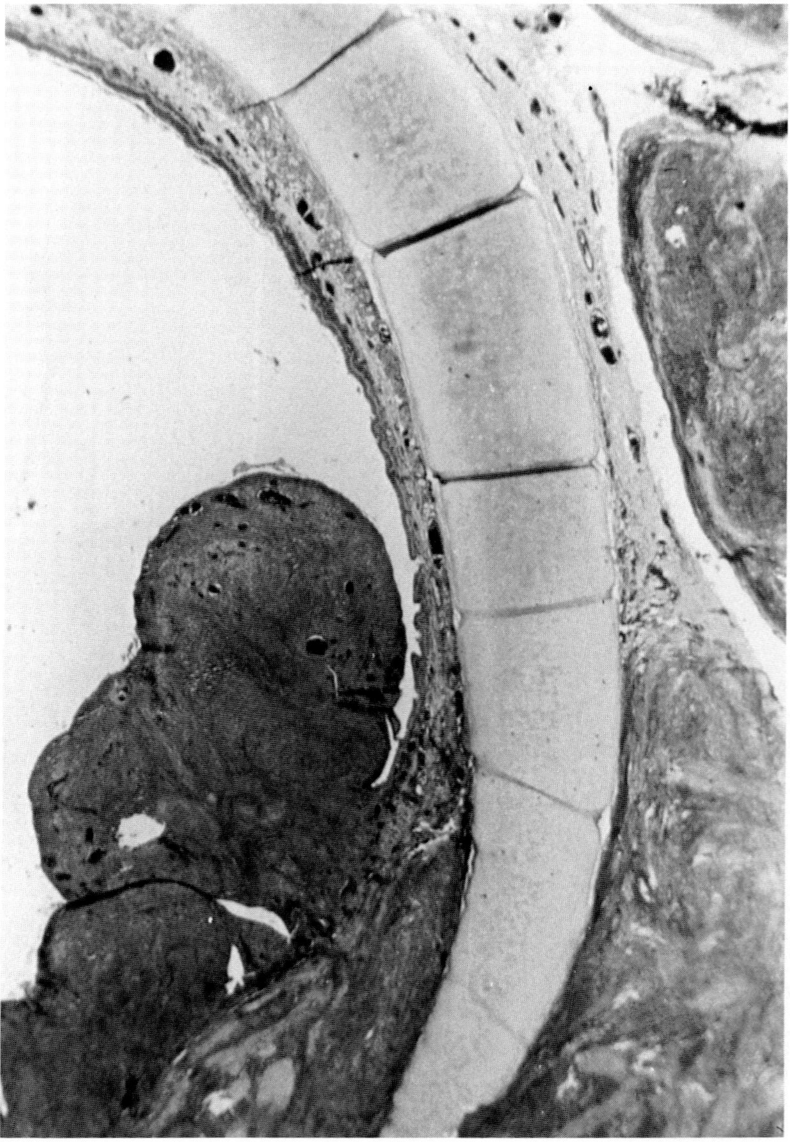

Figure 13 Endotracheal ulcerating tumor mass. Note the extensive infiltration in the peritracheal tissues.

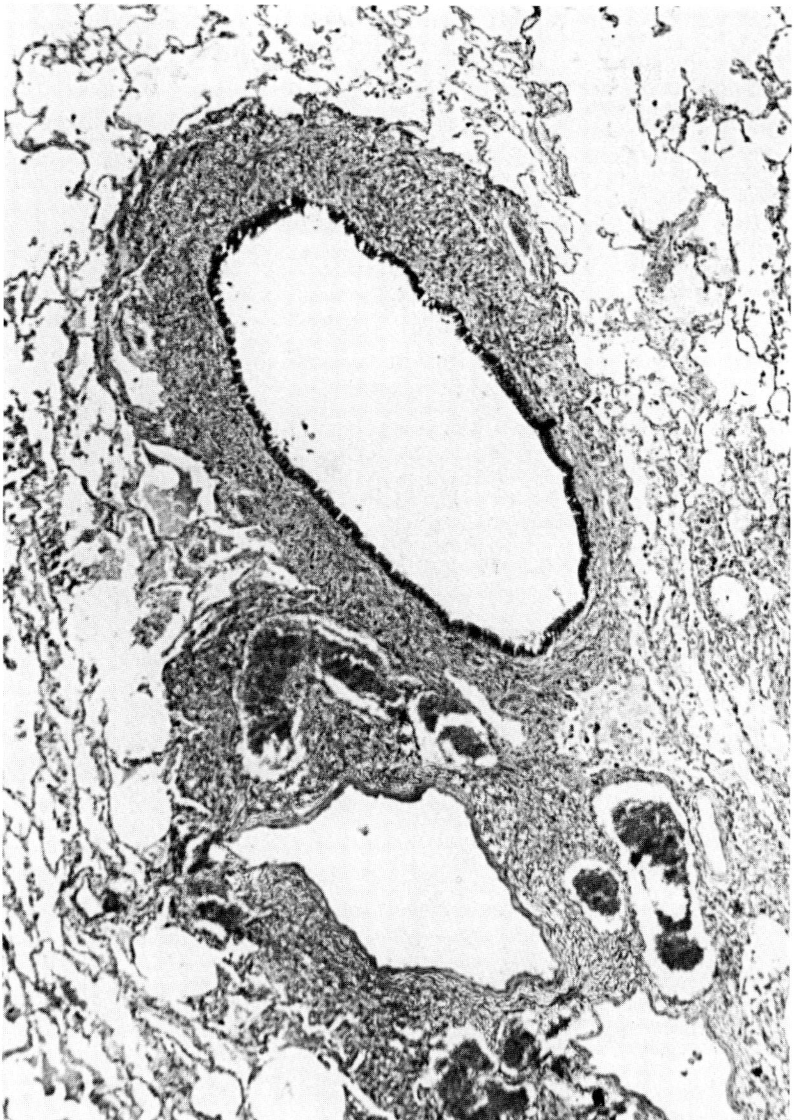

Figure 14 Characteristic peribronchial and perivascular mantle of tumor within the lung.

the diagnosis is usually only made by open biopsy or at autopsy. Lung biopsy interpretation is easiest when careful attention is paid to the low-power appearance. The thick mantle of tumor around the major vessels is very characteristic and is seldom mimicked even by lymphangitis carcinomatosum. The presence of a spindle cell proliferation etching along the pulmonary septa and sometimes extending into neighboring interstitium is characteristic and readily distinguishable from the appearance of adult respiratory distress syndrome or viral pneumonia. Recognition of parenchymal Kaposi's sarcoma on transbronchial biopsy in the absence of major airway disease may be difficult because the volume of tissue obtained is usually small. Fortunately, this is an unusual circumstance since most patients with parenchymal tumors also show at least a few plaques recognizable by the experienced endoscopist. If the pathologist actively seeks a mantle of cells around the largest bronchus or vessel in the biopsy and then looks for spindle cells within this, then the diagnosis can be made in a high proportion of cases (47). This proportion is bound to rise as familiarity with this pattern of disease increases. Current practice in the diagnosis of pulmonary complications of AIDS is shifting away from biopsy, toward the use of bronchial lavage since this procedure carries less risk of complications and is quite accurate in the diagnosis of infection. This will tend to cause an underdiagnosis of Kaposi's sarcoma, since in most cases there is no exfoliation of tumor cells in the absence of ulceration of the bronchial mucosa. The diagnosis of Kaposi's sarcoma can be suspected on a lavage specimen when iron-containing macrophages are seen in an immunodeficient host who is not in heart failure (44).

Lymph Nodes

Lymph node enlargement is seen in many patients with Kaposi's sarcoma. In patients with the classic nodular pattern it is usually reactive and shows the features of dermatopathic lymphadenopathy. In rare cases an isolated node may be replaced by Kaposi's sarcoma, and such patients have been cured by its removal (personal observation). Locally aggressive lesions may show involvement of nodes in a fashion identical to that seen in metastasis from epithelial tumors, that is, involvement of the peripheral sinus and gradual encroachment in the node thereafter (Figure 15).

The childhood lymphadenopathic form shows widespread nodal involvement by definition. In this form of Kaposi's sarcoma, the nodes show permeation of virtually every sinus in virtually every node by a spindle cell and vascular proliferation. Larger nodules form at scattered points, and at the time of presentation, the tumor usually occupies about 90% of the volume of any node (Figure 16). In AIDS-related disease nodal involvement may be identified in a high proportion of cases; estimates vary from 30 to 95% (37). The true incidence is probably closer to the latter figure. Involvement of the lymph node by Kaposi's sarcoma may be extremely subtle. The pattern is that of a gradual expansion of the sinuses by a combination of vascular and spindle cell proliferation, which then impinges on adjacent tissue to form the classic nodular pattern. It is particularly easy to miss the diagnosis when some other disease, such as mycobacterial infection or lymphoma, is present. In many sections only a fine mantle of spindle cells along the sinus gives a clue to the diagnosis. Serial sections of such nodes often reveal a nodular area where the diagnosis can be made with confidence. In its early stages Kaposi's sarcoma strongly resembles the changes in congested nodes, the so-called vascular transformation of nodal sinuses.

This much is universally agreed upon by all authorities. Some (37,48,49) have sought to expand the definition of Kaposi's sarcoma to include a lymphoid and vascular proliferation, which does not fulfill the classic criteria for diagnosis of Kaposi's sarcoma but is often seen in the same node as with the classic nodular pattern. This has been called the inflammatory form of the disease (37). This proliferation could also be interpreted as a reactive change that precedes the development of Kaposi's sarcoma rather than representing morphologically distinct phases of the same disease.

Malignant lymphoma and Kaposi's sarcoma occur together in a greater than random frequency. Hodgkin's disease, diffuse lympho-

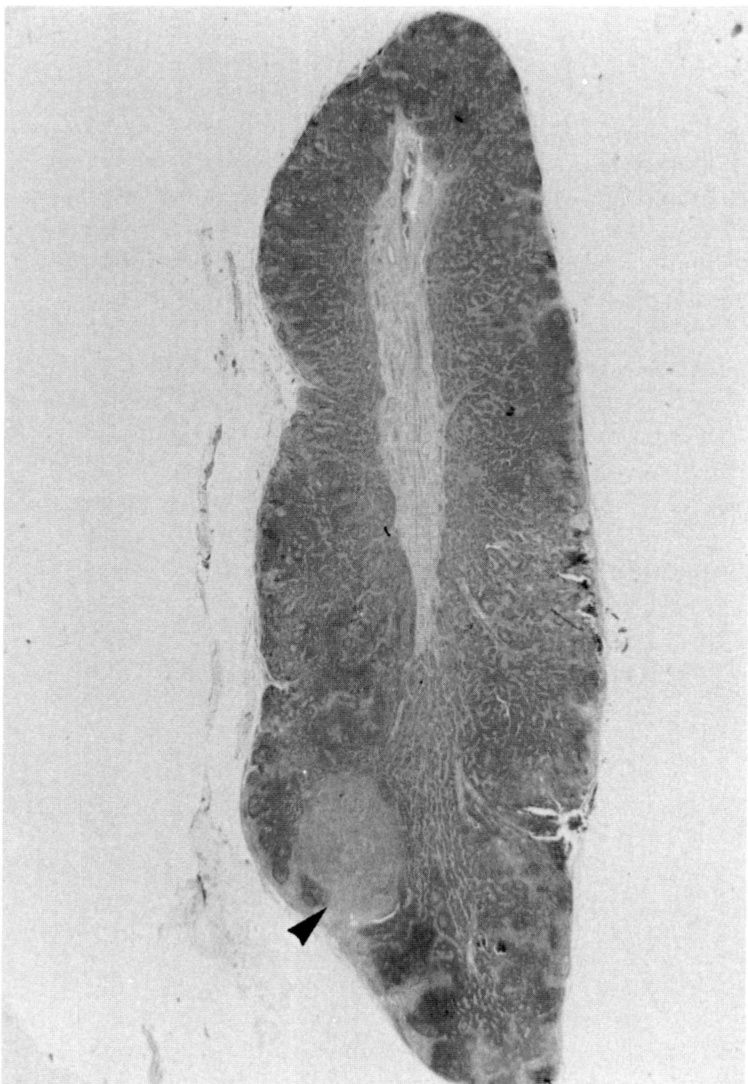

Figure 15 Low-power view of a lymph node invaded by metastasis from a locally aggressive tumor on the foot. Note involvement of the peripheral sinus in one part of the node only (arrow). Adjacent sinuses show sinus hyperplasia but there is no tumor.

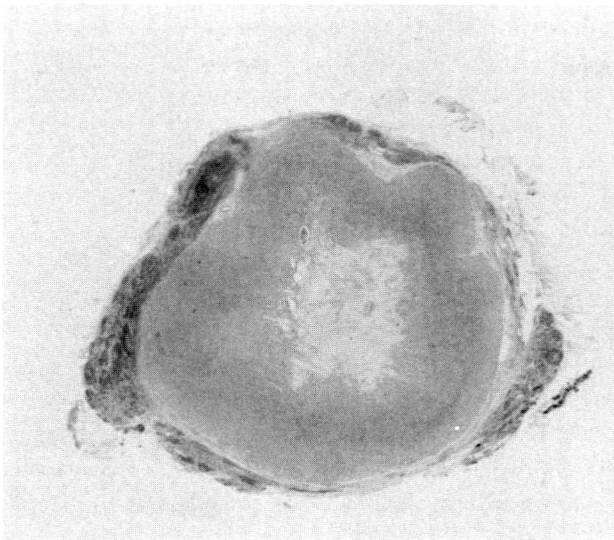

Figure 16 Lymph node from an African child with generalized lymph node enlargement with a centrally placed nodule with residual nodal tissue around it.

cytic lymphoma, and leukemia have all been described in patients with Kaposi's sarcoma, often in the same node. Most authorities regard this association as indirect, although transitional forms are described (50). This author's opinion is that virally induced inflammation, malignant lymphoma, and Kaposi's sarcoma, although statistically linked, are separate and separable entities even if the development of one facilitates the other. Which is not to say that the distinctions are easy to make. Whichever one believes, lymph nodes in AIDS are seldom normal. At different stages of the disease they may show follicular hyperplasia or depopulation. Fibrosis and/or vascular proliferation are seen particularly in African and Haitian subjects. A wide variety of infections produce nodal changes. It is within such a background that Kaposi's sarcoma develops in the AIDS-associated disease. Kaposi's sarcoma has been described in association with just about every known lymph node perturbation from lymphoma to Castleman's disease, angioimmunoblastic lymphadenopathy, and tuberculosis. Thus early changes of Kaposi's sarcoma are often obscured by an overlay of inflammatory cells. With such difficulties in determining the early phases of the development of the disease, wide variations in the frequency statistics are anticipated.

Splenic Involvement

The spleen is virtually never involved in patients with classic nodular disease and is only rarely affected in patients with AIDS or in the generalized African form. An autopsy series composed predominantly of Haitian patients (37) showed a much higher incidence. This is at least partially explicable on the basis of differences of diagnostic criteria, but it may be that different epidemiologic groups show a different distribution of systemic involvement. When present, splenic involvement shows a pattern rather similar to that seen in the lung. Cords and strands of tumor appear to follow the major vessels out into the red pulp. Nodules per se are relatively rarely seen.

Skeletal Lesions

The bone marrow is rarely involved. Patients with locally aggressive disease quite commonly show involvement of adjacent bones either as a medullary expansion or as a cortical notching due to a periosteal tumor. Otherwise, involvement of the cortex or medulla of bone remote from subcutaneous sites of involvement is unusual.

Liver

Involvement of the liver usually follows the portal areas in a tendrillike fashion, and involvement of the sinusoids and parenchymal area is unusual. Such symptoms as jaundice or portal hypertension are only rarely seen.

Central Nervous System

Involvement of the central nervous system by Kaposi's sarcoma is rare. Scattered case reports have appeared at exactly 10-year intervals (51–55), but two of these (52,53) must be regarded with some suspicion as these patients did not have skin lesions. All the reported patients had extensive pulmonary disease, and it may be that this is an important risk factor. This would not be surprising, since many other pulmonary conditions, such as bronchiectasis and neoplasms, are associated with cerebral metastases.

Unusual Sites of Involvement

Other parts of the body are involved relatively infrequently. The pericardium may show many nodular deposits, but the myocardium is relatively rarely involved. The external genitalia show involvement in nodular disease, but the bladder, ureter, and gonads are very infrequently the site of lesions. Renal involvement is unusual, but when it occurs it follows the pattern very typical of parenchymal organs, with a sheath of tumor spreading out from the hilum along the path of arcuate vessels. Isolated nodules may be seen in the adrenal cortex, but involvement of the medulla or other endocrine glands has yet to be described.

SUMMARY

The classic mixture of spindle cells and capillary vascular spaces is faithfully recapitulated in the vast majority of lesions of patients with Kaposi's sarcoma regardless of the clinical pattern exhibited. This means that the diagnosis can be confidently made in most situations with paraffin sections stained with hematoxylin and eosin.

Difficulties are encountered in skin and lymph nodes, particularly at the interface of granulation tissue and in early lesions of Kaposi's sarcoma. The key observations that strengthen the diagnosis are presence of spindle cells, erythrophagocytosis, and clusters of eosinophilic inclusions in Kaposi's sarcoma and the presence of polymorphonuclear leukocytes in granulation tissue. In difficult cases electron microscopy is distinctive in that microscopic vessels within the tumor nodule show a lack of perithelial investment and an incomplete basement membrane.

Underneath mucosal or cutaneous surfaces, the tumor displays plaque to nodule progression with ulceration occurring late in the disease. In parenchymal organs, such as lung, liver, and kidney, the tumor adopts a sheathlike investment of major vessels and ducts, with nodules occurring infrequently. The rarity of involvement of the brain is confirmed, and this may relate to the lack of lymphatic channels at this site.

REFERENCES

1. Costa J, Rabson A. Generalized Kaposi's sarcoma is not a neoplasm. Lancet 1983; 1:58.
2. Bluefarb SM. Kaposi's sarcoma. Springfield, Illinois, Charles C. Thomas, 1957.
3. Templeton AC. Kaposi's sarcoma. In: Cancer of the Skin, Chapter 52, Andrade R, Gumport SC, Popkin GL, Rees TD, eds. Philadelphia, WB Saunders, 1976.
4. Taylor JF, Templeton AC, Vogel C, Ziegler JL, Kyalwazi SK. Kaposi's sarcoma in Uganda. A clinico-pathologic study, Int J Cancer 1971; 8:122–35.
5. Dutz W, Stout AP. Kaposi's sarcoma in infants and children. Cancer 1960 13:684–92.
6. Kusnezow WN. A case of sarcoma multiplex idiopathicum (Kaposi) with fatal outcome. Urol Cutan Rev 1933; 37:230–4.
7. Symmers D. Kaposi's sarcoma. Arch Pathol 1961; 32:764–7.
8. Collins MD, Fisher H. A case of generalized hemangiosarcomatosis erroneously considered as generalized tuberculosis. Am Rev Tuberc 1950; 61:257–9.
9. Hogeman O. Hyper hemolysis of non splenic origin. Acta Med Scand 1953; 144:247–50.

10. Reynolds WA, Winkelman RK, Soule EM. Kaposi's sarcoma. 1965; 44:419–43.
11. Safai B, Johnson KG, Myskowski DL, Koziner B, Yang SY, Cunningham-Rundles S, Dupont B. The natural history of Kaposi's sarcoma in the acquired immunodeficiency syndrome. Ann Intern Med 1985; 103:744–50.
12. Mitsuyasu RT, Taylor JMG, Glaspy J, Fahey JL. Heterogeneity of epidemic Kaposi's sarcoma. Implications for therapy. Cancer 1986; 57:1657–61.
13. Francis ND, Parkin JM, Weber J, Boylston AW. Kaposi's sarcoma in acquired immune deficiency syndrome (AIDS). J Clin Pathol 1986; 39:469–74.
14. Serwadda D, Carswell W, Ayudho WO, Wanusota W, Madda P, Downing RG. Further experience with Kaposi's sarcoma in Uganda. Br J Cancer 1986; 53:497–500.
15. Russell Jones R, Spaull J, Spry C, Wilson Jones E. Histogenesis of Kaposi's sarcoma in patients with and without acquired immunodeficiency syndrome (AIDS). J Clin Pathol 1986; 39:742–9.
16. Leu HJ, Odermatt B. Multicentric angiosarcoma. Light and electron-microscopic and immunohistological findings of idiopathic cases in Europe and Africa and of cases associated with AIDS. Virchows Arch (Pathol Anat) 1985; 408:29–41.
17. Modlin RL, Hofman FM, Kempf RA, Taylor CR, Conant MA, Rea TM. Kaposi's sarcoma in homosexual men: an immunohistochemical study. J Am Acad Dermatol 1983; 8:620–7.
18. Blumenfeld W, Egbert BM, Sagebiel RW. Differential diagnosis of Kaposi's sarcoma. Arch Pathol Lab Med 1985; 109:123–7.
19. Ackerman AB. Subtle clues to diagnosis by conventional microscopy. The Patch stage of Kaposi's sarcoma. Am J Dermatopathol 1979; 1:165–72.
20. Schwartz JL, Muhlbauer JE, Steigbigel RT. Pre Kaposi's sarcoma. Am Acad Dermatol 1984; 11:377–80.
21. Green TL, Beckstead JM, Lozada Nur F, Silverman S, Hansen LS. Histopathologic spectrum of oral Kaposi's sarcoma. Oral Surg 1984; 58:306–14.
22. McNutt NS, Fletcher V, Conant MA. Early lesions of Kaposi's sarcoma in homosexual men. An ultrastructural comparison with other vascular proliferations in skin. Am J Pathol 1983; 111:62–77.
23. Freedman-Kien AE, Laubenstein LJ, Rubinstein P. Disseminated

Kaposi's sarcoma in homosexual men. Ann Intern Med 1982; 96: 693–700.
24. Penneys NS, Hicks B. Unusual cutaneous lesions associated with acquired immunodeficiency syndrome. J Am Acad Dermatopathol 1985; 13:845–52.
25. Weiss SW, Enzinger FM. Spindle cell hemangioendothelioma. A low grade angiosarcoma resembling a cavernous hemangioma and Kaposi's sarcoma. Am J Surg Pathol 1986; 10:521–30.
26. Hashimoto H, Daimaru Y, Enjoji M. Intravascular papillary endothelial hyperplasia. A clinicopathologic study of 91 cases. Am J Dermatopathol 1983; 5:539–46.
27. Reed CN, Cooper TM, Swerlick RA. Intravascular papillary endothelial hyperplasia. J Am Acad Dermatol 1984; 10:110–3.
28. Kuo T, Gomez LG. Papillary endothelial proliferation in cystic lymphangioma. Arch Pathol Lab Med 1979; 103:306–8.
29. Mali JWH, Kuiper JP, Hamers AA. Acroangiodermatitis of the foot. Arch Dermatol 1965; 92:515–8.
30. Goldblum OM, Kraus E, Bronner AK. Pseudo-Kaposi's sarcoma of the hand associated with an acquired iatrogenic fistula. Arch Dermatol 1985; 121:1038–40.
31. Schamroth JM, Ratanjee H, Kellen P, Jaques V, Leibowitz M. Kaposi's sarcoma localized to the site of previous vascular surgery. Arch Dermatol 1985; 121:969–70.
32. Secher L, Weismann K, Kobayasi T. Pseudo-Kaposi's sarcoma of the feet: an electron microscopic investigation. Acta Derm Venereol (Stockh) 1984; 64:246–9.
33. Weldon Linne CM, Rhone DP, Blatt D, Moore D, Monitz M. Angiolipomas in homosexual males. N Engl J Med 1984; 310:1193.
34. Santa Cruz DJ, Kyriachos M. Aneurysmal (angiomatoid) fibrous histiocytoma of the skin. Cancer 1981; 47:2053–61.
35. Enzinger FM. Angiomatoid malignant fibrous histiocytoma. Cancer 1979; 46:2147–57.
36. Waldo E, Stahl R, Sidmu GS, Zolla-Pazner S. Histiocytoid hemangioma with features of angiolymphoid hyperplasia and Kaposi's sarcoma. Am J Dermatopathol 1983; 5:525–38.
37. Moskowitz EB, Hensley,GT, Gould EW, Weiss SD. Frequency and anatomic distribution of lymphadenopathic Kaposi's sarcoma in the acquired immunodeficiency syndrome. Hum Pathol 1985; 6:447–56.
38. Bernal A, delJunco GW, Gibson SR. Endoscopic and pathologic

features of gastrointestinal Kaposi's sarcoma. Gastrointest Endosc 1985; 31:74–7.
39. Friedman SL, Wright TL, Altman DF. Gastrointestinal Kaposi's sarcoma in patient's with acquired immunodeficiency syndrome. Endoscopic and autopsy findings. Gastroenterology 1985; 89:102–8.
40. Saltz RK, Kurtz RC, Lightdale CJ, Myskowski P, Cunningham-Rundles S, Urmacher C, Safai B. Kaposi's sarcoma. Gastrointestinal involvement, correlation with skin findings and immunologic function. Dig Dis Sci 1984; 29:817–23.
41. Mitchell N, Feder T. Kaposi's sarcoma with secondary involvement of the jejunum, perforation and peritonitis. Ann Intern Med 1949; 31:324–9.
42. Meduri GU, Stover DE, Lee M, Myskowski PL, Caravelli JF, Zaman MB. Pulmonary Kaposi's sarcoma in the acquired immune deficiency syndrome. Clinical, radiographic and pathologic manifestations. Am J Med 1986; 81:11–8.
43. Nash G, Fligiel S. Kaposi's sarcoma presenting as pulmonary disease in the acquired immunodeficiency syndrome. Diagnosis by lung biopsy. Hum Pathol 1984; 15:999–1001.
44. Touboul JL, Mayaud CM, Fouret P, Akoun GM. Pulmonary lesions of Kaposi's sarcoma. Intra-alveolar hemorrhage and pleural effusion. Ann Intern Med 1985; 103:808.
45. Ognibene FP, Steis RG, Macher AM. Kaposi's sarcoma causing pulmonary infiltrate and respiratory failure in the acquired immune deficiency syndrome. Ann Intern Med 1985; 102:471–5.
46. Jollenberg JE, Fischl MA, Berger JR. Upper airway obstruction secondary to acquired immunodeficiency syndrome related Kaposi's sarcoma. Chest 1985; 88:638–40.
47. Purdy LJ, Colby TV, Yousem SA, Battifora H. Pulmonary Kaposi's sarcoma: Premortem histologic diagnosis. Am J Surg Pathol 1986; 10:301–11.
48. Rywlin AM, Rosen L, Cabello B. Coexistence of Castleman's disease and Kaposi's sarcoma. Am J Dermatopathol 1983; 5:277–81.
49. Amazon K, Rywlin AM. Subtle clues to diagnosis by conventional microscopy. Lymphnode involvement in Kaposi's sarcoma. Am J Dermatopathol 1979; 1:173–6.
50. Uys CJ, Bennett MD. Kaposi's sarcoma accurring in a coloured male. S Afr Med J 1958; 32:577–81.
51. Nesbitt S, Mark PF, Zimmerman HM. Disseminated visceral hemor-

rhagic sarcoma (Kaposi's disease). Report of a case with necropsy findings. Ann Intern Med 1945; 22:601–5.
52. Schirrin CG, Burkhardt L. Ein sarcoma idiopathicum multiplex hemorrhagicum (Kaposi) mit Shirn Metastasen. Arch Klin Exp Dermatol 1955; 201:99.
53. Loring WF, Woleman SR. Idiopathic multiple hemorrhagic sarcoma of lung. (Kaposi's sarcoma). NY State J Med 1965; 65:668–76.
54. Rwamushana RJW, Bailey TC, Kyalwazi SK. Kaposi's sarcoma of the Brain. Cancer 1975; 36:1127–31.
55. Garin FA, Bale JF, Halks-Miller M, Schwartz RA. Kaposi's sarcoma metastatic to the CNS. Arch Neurol 1985; 42:162–5.

3

Histogenesis

Ronald F. Dorfman
Stanford University Medical Center
Stanford, California

Gary S. Wood
Stanford University Medical Center
Stanford, California
and Veterans Administration Medical Center
Palo Alto, California

Jay H. Beckstead
University of California
San Francisco, California

Although 114 years have elapsed since Kaposi (1) described the disorder that bears his name, the etiology and histogenesis of this condition remain a subject of controversy. Hypotheses on the nature and origin of the spindle cell of Kaposi's sarcoma were initially based largely on morphological observations, supported to some extent by the correlation with clinical behavior and course of the disease. Subsequently, such methods as enzyme histochemistry and electron microscopy were applied to the study of Kaposi's sarcoma and attempts were made to establish cell lines in tissue culture and to reproduce the disease experimentally in animals. In 1975, Kohler and Milstein succeeded in immortalizing antibody production and in developing monoclonal antibodies (MoAB) (2). During the next decade MoAB would prove to be a basic tool in studies of cell surface antigens in normal and neoplastic cells, and a number of these MoAB have been applied to the study of Kaposi's sarcoma. The role of such viruses as cytomegalovirus (CMV) (3), herpes simplex (HSV) (4), Epstein-Barr virus (EBV) (5), and the lymphotropic retroviruses HTLV-III/LAV (6,7) (now termed human immunodeficiency virus, HIV) (8), as etiologic agents is currently under intense scrutiny. Moreover, it has become evident that immunosuppression plays an important role in the pathogenesis of Kaposi's sarcoma, at least in transplant recipients (9–11) and in association with the acquired immunodeficiency syndrome (AIDS) (12,13). We shall explore and discuss theories of the histogenesis of Kaposi's sarcoma based on the results of these studies.

MORPHOLOGIC OBSERVATIONS AT THE LIGHT MICROSCOPIC LEVEL

In 1961, Dorfman had the privilege of attending the symposium on Kaposi's sarcoma held at Makerere Medical College, Kampala, Uganda, under the auspices of the Union Internationale Contre Le Cancer (International Union Against Cancer) (14). There was much speculation concerning the histogenesis of the cellular components of Kaposi's sarcoma, particularly the spindle cell. Roulet

(15) favored a vascular neoformation in which the entire wall of the capillary appeared to participate in the proliferative process. Murray and Lothe (16) expressed their belief that Kaposi's sarcoma was a malignant neoplasm of multicentric origin and that it originated from the region of the adventitia of the blood vessels, possibly from undifferentiated mesenchymal cells, Schwann cells, or pericytes. Although emphasizing that there was little to be gained by tedious reiteration of the various arguments put forward by different observers in support of their hypotheses, Becker (17) nonetheless noted that indirect evidence had been advanced for origin from the following cellular sources: reticuloendothelial system (18–21); primitive mesenchymal cell (22); neuromyoarterial apparatus (23–25); blood vascular endothelium (19,20,26–29); lymph vascular endothelium (20,29,30); fibroblasts (31); smooth muscle (32); perithelial cells (33–35); and combined endothelial and perithelial cells (36). Becker (17) indicated that, based on his own observations and those of Pepler (37), Kaposi's sarcoma always arises from a perivascular or immediately perivascular site and the likely cellular source of this tumor is the perivascular Schwann cell.

In a recently published report, Dorfman (38) quoted from the writings of Arthur Purdy Stout (39), who cited reports of others postulating "a malformation of vessels and nerves, akin to multiple neurofibromatosis, and an angiomatosis with new formation of vessels of the neuromyoarterial glomus type, vasculo-nervous elements and Schwann cells." Stout himself appeared to favor the concept of an "angiosarcomatosis," describing Kaposi's sarcoma as a complex vascular growth consisting of capillaries and fibrosarcoma-like cells in symbiosis. He expressed uncertainty about whether this was a true neoplastic process but commented that "it seems impossible to avoid reference to it in any consideration of malignant vascular tumors."

The problem of the histogenesis of spindle cells in Kaposi's sarcoma has interested investigators as far back as 1899, when Schwimmer (30) suggested an origin from lymphatic endothelial cells. Lothe and Murray (40), participants at the Kampala symposium in 1961, emphasized the predominant localization of lesions in the lymphatic system in African children and the striking distribution of lesions around blood vessels, often in the form of thick strands of tumor tissue extending around the outer walls of the vessels for a considerable distance. The distribution could be seen by the naked eye to follow the portal tracts in the liver and histologically to be closely associated with branching blood vessels in the spleen and in the lung. The situation of these lesions was considered to be in keeping with their origin from lymphatics, which are present in the outer coat of blood vessels. Tumor tissue was also seen around nerve fibers and along the lines of lymphatics in the limbs. The striking absence of lesions in the brain and in the eyeball, in cases encountered in Uganda and southern Africa, was emphasized, and it was noted that these organs are devoid of lymphatics, apart from small capillaries following the course of blood vessels and cranial nerves (41).

It was suggested that the various hemodynamic disturbances exhibited by some patients with Kaposi's sarcoma could be explained on the basis of lymphaticovenous anastomoses. Such lesions were in fact demonstrated by Palmer (42) during the Kampala conference. It was therefore postulated by Dorfman (43) that multicentric neoformation of lymphatics is a primary process in the histogenesis of Kaposi's sarcoma, that the predominant localization of lesions corresponds to the normal distribution of lymphatics, and that the pathological formation of lymphaticovenous anastomoses could account for the many clinical manifestations of Kaposi's sarcoma.

Some 25 years later Dictor (44), after a review of histopathological material from 9 autopsies and 35 skin biopsy specimens of Kaposi's sarcoma in male homosexuals, indicated that aberrant lymphaticovenous connections occur in the earliest stage of Kaposi's sarcoma. Dictor proposed that the initiation of the lesion may be an abnormal recapitulation of the coupling of venous and lymphatic sinuses that occurs during embryonic growth. Although recognizing that the precise origin of the characteristic spindle cells in the developing lesion remains unclear, he suggested that convergent differentiation of lymphatic and blood vascular endothelium may be considered. He also commented that microcirculation, particularly that distal to the capillary bed, may explain several of the histopathological and hemodynamic features of Kaposi's sarcoma, including lesional thrombosis and infarction, tissue hemorrhage, vascular dilatation, cavernous pseudoangiomas, and acute right-sided heart failure.

In our own studies on lesions of Kaposi's sarcoma in skin and in lymph nodes (45), we have noted a pattern of development suggestive of lymphatic origin (see Figures 1 through 8). The earliest lesions consist of irregular thin-walled vascular spaces lined by plump endothelial cells morphologically suggestive of lymphatics (Figures 1 through 3). These vascular structures surround and separate preexisting collagen bundles, vessels, and nerves to form a distinctive spongy network (Figures 3 and 4). In lesions in which these spaces are not dilated they are more difficult to identify. In more advanced lesions, the picture is complicated by neovascularization, producing distinctive structures with a core composed of a morphologically and phenotypically normal capillary, venule, or arteriole, a modest amount of collagen, and moderate numbers of inflammatory cells, covered by layers of proliferating abnormal endothelial cells (Figures 4 and 5). With further proliferation, the abnormal endothelial cells accumulate and occasionally form solid cords (Figures 6 and 7). The vascular cores also proliferate, apparently in response to the tumor. This proliferation produces very vascular lesions in which the abnormal endothelium may be difficult to distinguish from the reactive normal vessels. Continued proliferation of the abnormal endothelial cells ultimately overwhelms the other elements, which results in solid sheets of spindle cells (Figures 7 and 8). Inflammatory cells, particularly macrophages, are frequently intermixed.

Several observers at the Kampala conference drew attention to the presence of spherical, homogenous globules or inclusions (intracellular or intercellular) associated with the spindle cells of Kaposi's sarcoma (16,46). In 1968, Lee (47) considered these "hyaline bodies" to be useful in the differential diagnosis of Kaposi's sarcoma and particularly in its differentiation from granuloma

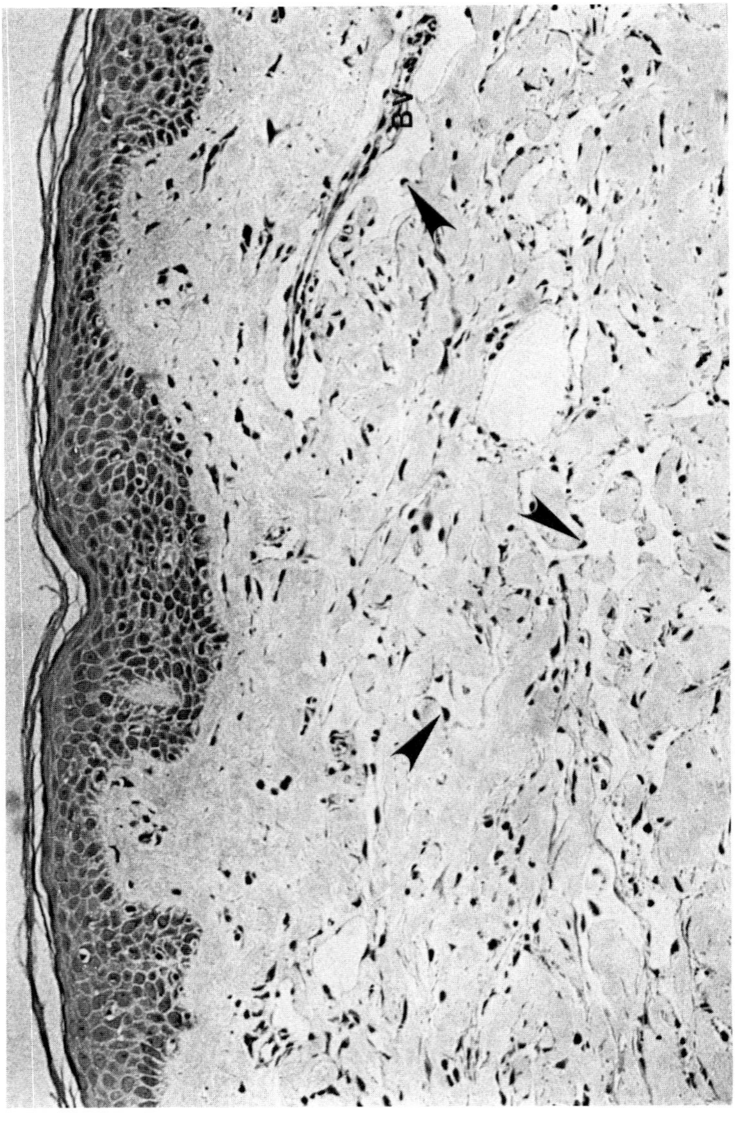

Figure 1 Early lesion of Kaposi's sarcoma in the skin. Irregular vascular spaces (arrows) lined by slightly plump endothelial cells are present within the dermis. They dissect bundles of collagen and frequently isolate preexisting structures, particularly blood vessels (BV). (Plastic section, H&E, ×160)

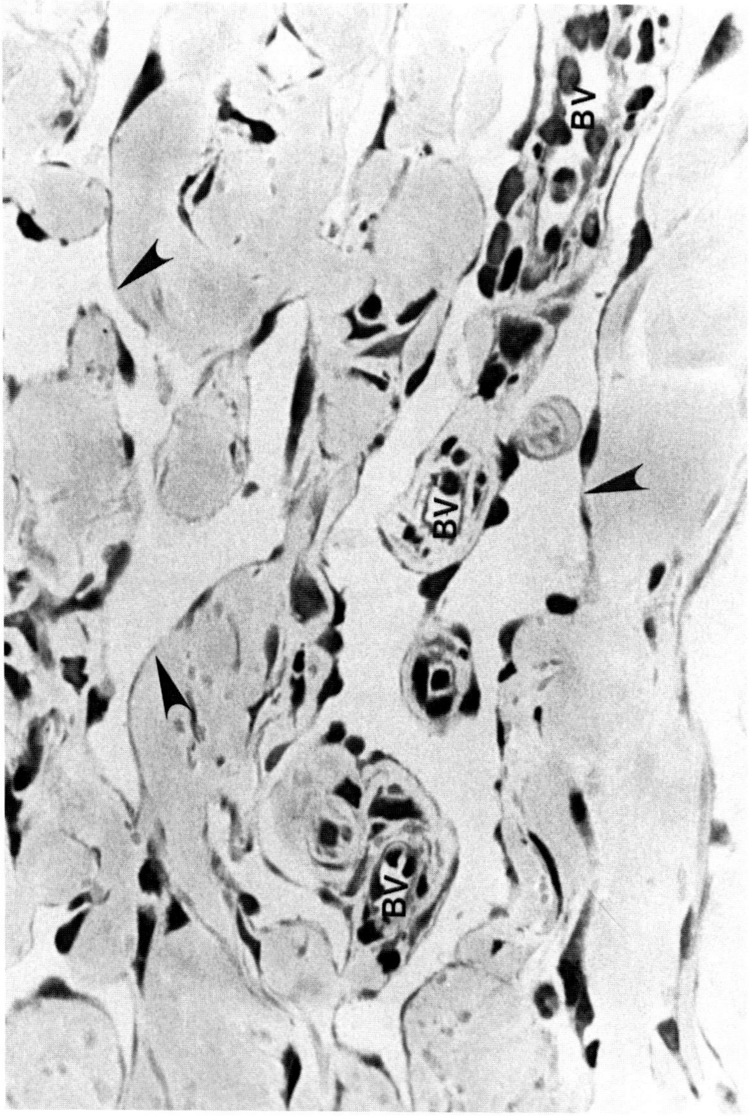

Figure 2 Early lesion of Kaposi's sarcoma in the skin. The endothelial nature of the spaces is more apparent at higher magnification. Normal blood vessels (BV) are surrounded and isolated by the abnormal vascular channels (arrows) lined by endothelial cells. (Plastic section, H&E, ×640)

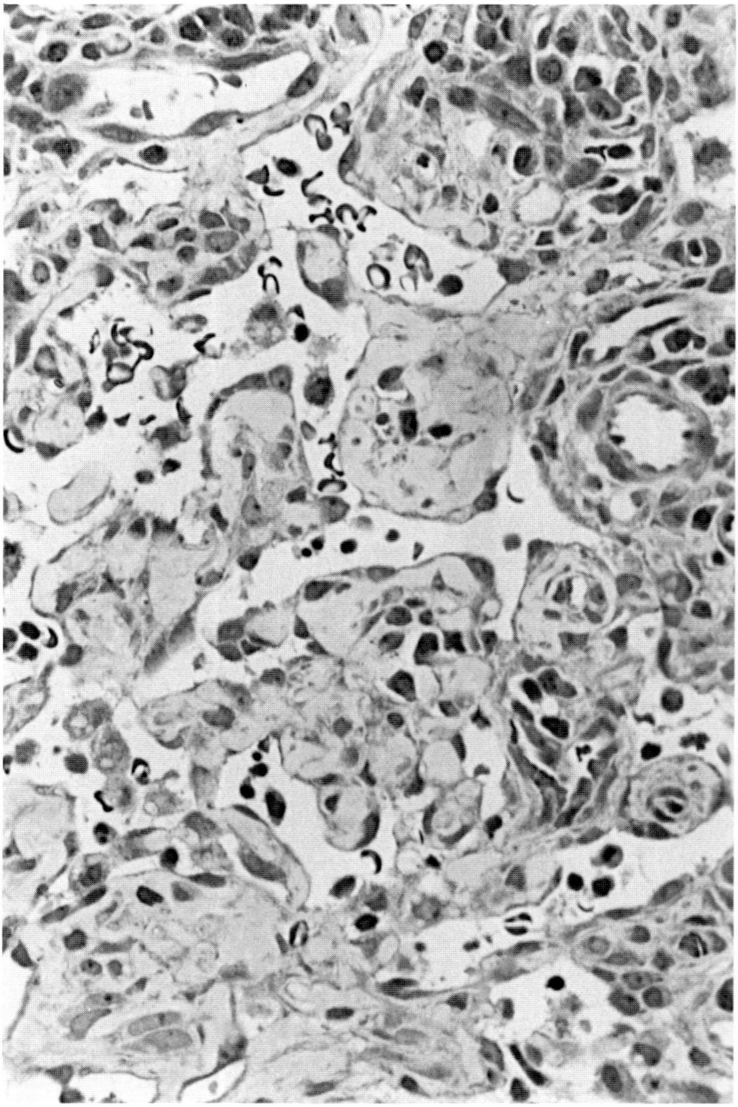

Figure 3 Early Kaposi's sarcoma in a lymph node. Irregular vascular spaces are also formed in lymph nodes. (Plastic section, H&E, ×400)

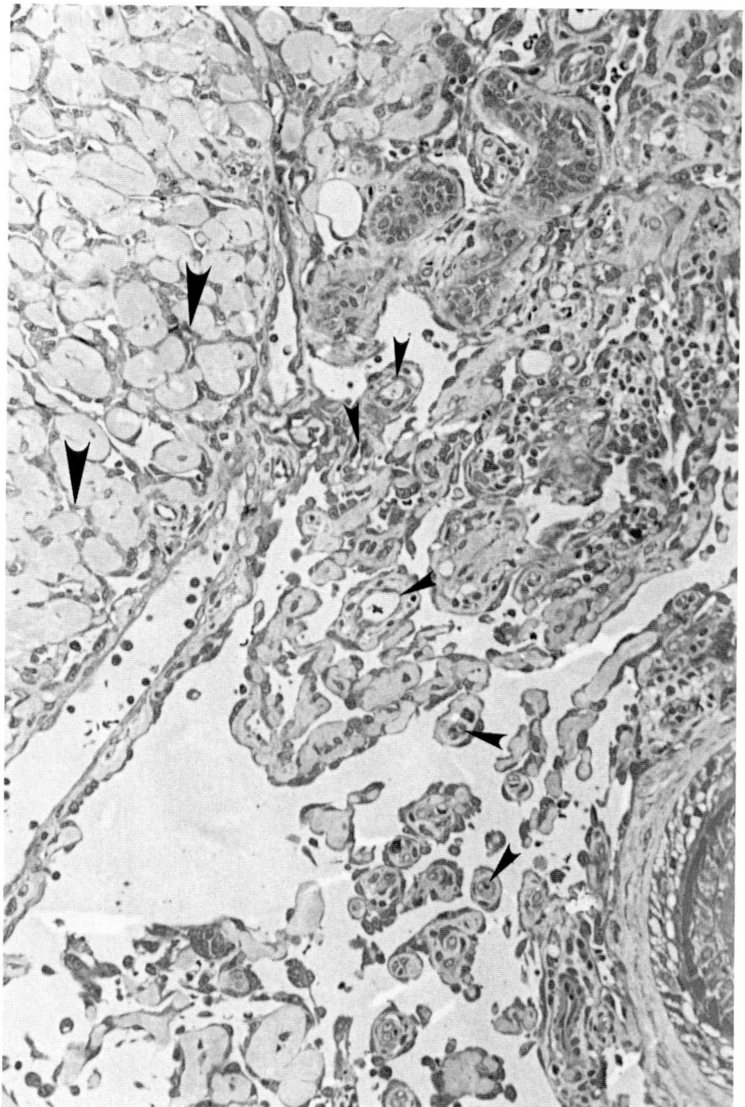

Figure 4 Kaposi's sarcoma in the skin. The proliferation of irregular vascular channels is more complex here, and the endothelial cells are slightly atypical. Normal blood vessels (small arrows) are present within many of the isolated bundles of collagen. In other areas (large arrows) the spaces are collapsed and less obvious. (Plastic section, H&E, ×160)

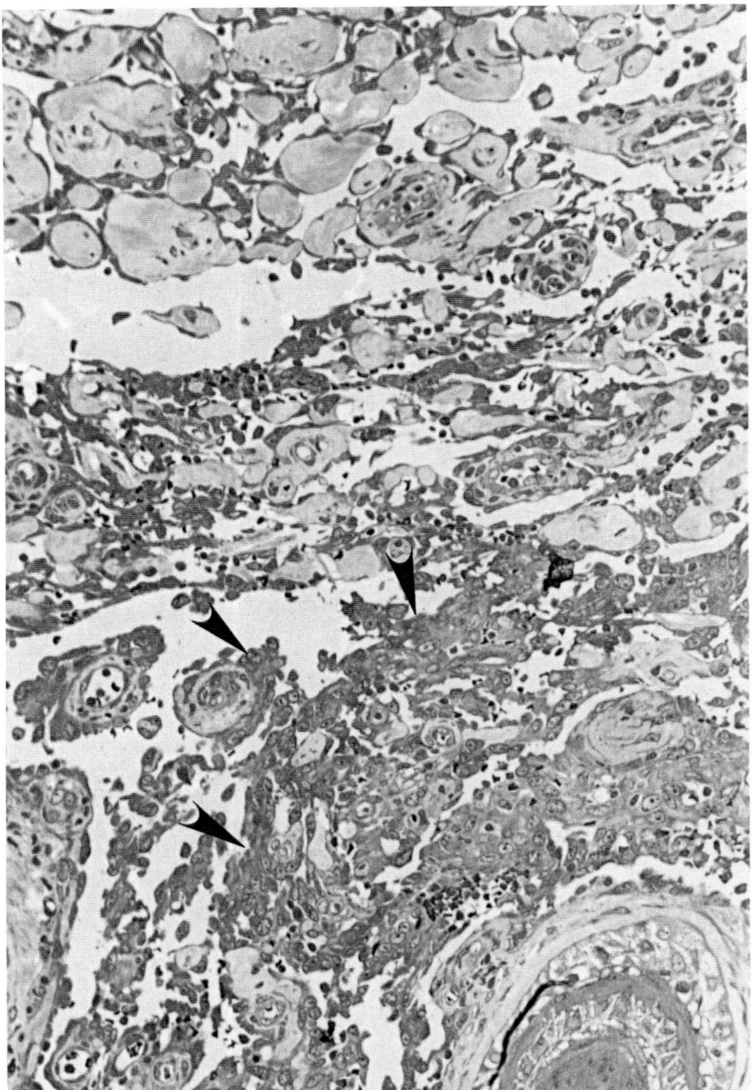

Figure 5 Kaposi's sarcoma in the skin. As the abnormal cells proliferate they begin to pile up (arrows). (Plastic section, H&E, ×160)

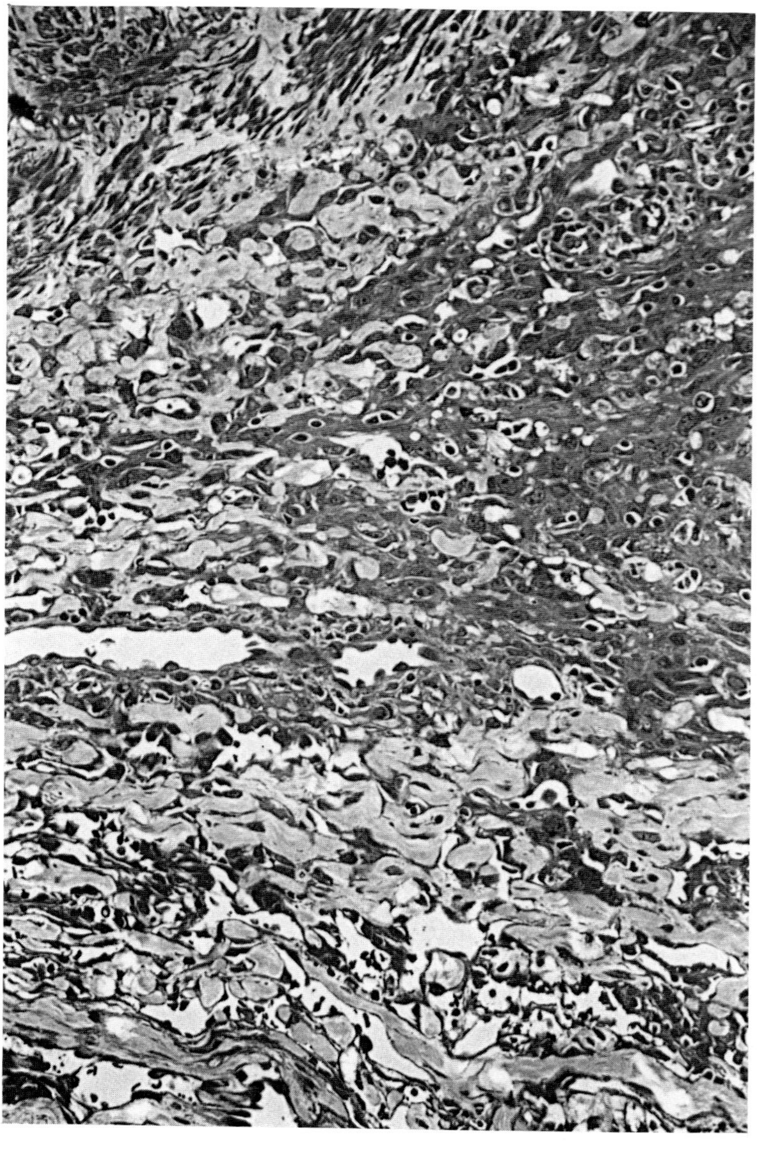

Figure 6 Kaposi's sarcoma in the skin. Continued proliferation obscures the abnormal spaces and the cells become more spindle shaped. (Plastic section, H&E, ×160)

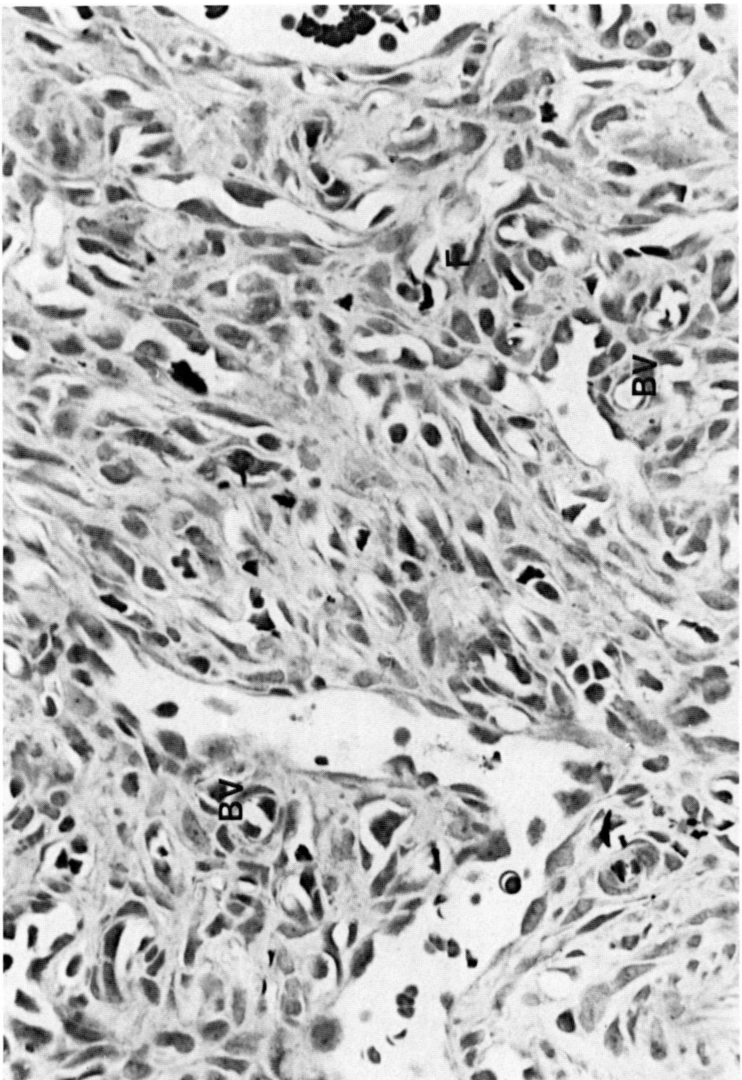

Figure 7 Kaposi's sarcoma in a lymph node. Continued proliferation tends to obscure the abnormal spaces and the relationship to normal blood vessels (BV). (Plastic section, H&E, ×400)

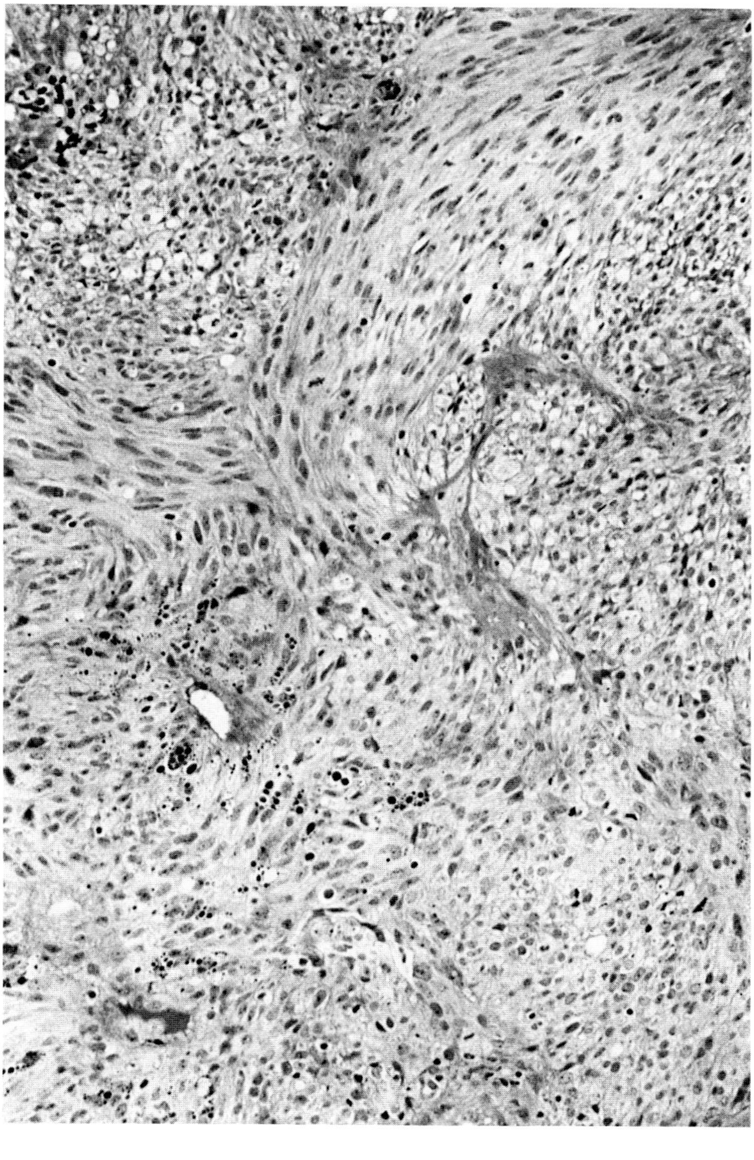

Figure 8 Kaposi's sarcoma in a lymph node. As the lesions progress the proliferating spindle cells crowd out the other normal and abnormal components of the early lesions. (Plastic section, H&E, ×160)

pyogenicum. These globules often appear to lie within macrophages (48). They resemble small Russell bodies and appear as dense osmiophilic bodies in the electron microscope. As discussed by Lee (47) and subsequently by Templeton (49), they may represent the products of lysosomal degeneration or effete red cells. Whatever their nature, they present a useful marker for Kaposi's sarcoma, particularly in its distinction from granuloma pyogenicum.

No better review of Kaposi's sarcoma is available prior to 1957 than that in Bluefarb's book (50), which contains a comprehensive bibliography on histogenetic concepts based on light microscopic and morbid anatomic observations.

MORPHOLOGIC OBSERVATIONS AT THE ELECTRON MICROSCOPIC LEVEL

The earliest reported electron microscopic study of Kaposi's sarcoma appears to be that of Pepler and Theron (51), who concluded that the tumor cell cytoplasm contained laminated structures resembling axis cylinders enclosed in membranes. Moreover, continuity could be established between the superficial plasma membrane and the membranous layers of the intracytoplasmic structures. They also noted that the tumor cells were surrounded by distinct basement membranes. They concluded therefore that the morphological features conformed with an origin of the tumor from Schwann cells. Subsequently, Hashimoto and Lever (52) indicated that the membranous structures described by Pepler and Theron and interpreted by them as schwannian myelin sheaths represented residual bodies of lysosomes (termed by some myelin bodies, to add to the confusion). Niemi and Mustakallio (53) made similar observations, indicating that the intracytoplasmic bodies were unlikely to represent myelin of nerve fibers but in all probability were the results of erythrophagocytosis in the spindle cells of Kaposi's sarcoma. Hashimoto and Lever (52) favored the concept that the tumor cells originated from pluripotential vascular cells, which gave rise to two main cell types composing the tumor, that is, endothelial cells and fibroblasts, actively engaged in the phagocytosis of extrasavated erythrocytes. Niemi and Mustakallio (53) presented similar views. Harrison and Kahn (54) summarized the results of seven reported ultrastructural studies indicating that endothelial cells were identified in six, fibroblasts in five, perithelial cells in three, histiocytes in two, mesenchymal cells in one, and smooth muscle in one. They emphasized that all these studies demonstrated either two or three cell types within an individual tumor.

The multiplicity of cell types and the presence of shared ultrastructural features suggested to several authors that the tumor was derived from a primitive pluripotential cell. In their own reported study, Harrison and Kahn (54) similarly identified the presence of endothelial cells, smooth muscle cells, fibroblasts and, in addition, myofibroblasts. They noted that some of these cells exhibited phagocytic activity related to extravasated red blood cells. They concluded that the ultrastructural features favored an origin of Kaposi's sarcoma from pluripotential mesenchymal cells that may differentiate into more specialized cell types, including endothelial, smooth muscle, fibroblastic, and myofibroblastic cells. Based on their observation of "infrequent Weibel-Palade bodies in tumor cells lining lumina," Waldo et al. (55) favored an endothelial cell differentiation.

In 1964, Dorfman (56) carried out an ultrastructural study of biopsies from three black African patients and three white American patients with Kaposi's sarcoma. Although the ultrastructural characteristics of spindle cells did not allow exact histogenetic identification, the occasional observation of zones of transition from identifiable endothelium to spindle cells, the presence of basement membranes, and the obvious clefts containing erythrocytes were considered consistent with the hypothesis that the spindle cells represented neoplastic endothelial cells. Distinction between lymphatic and blood vascular endothelium could not be made.

Recently, McNutt et al. (57) reported their ultrastructural observations in early lesions of Kaposi's sarcoma in homosexual men and compared these with other vascular proliferations in skin. They noted that in all cases of Kaposi's sarcoma, the small blood vessels lacked a prominent investment of pericytes, and their processes (observations confirmed by others; see Reference 58) had a fragmented and often absent basal lamina and showed frequent discontinuities in the endothelial lining and only a few small junctional densities between endothelial cells. Some clinically aggressive cases of Kaposi's sarcoma also showed necrosis of individual endothelial cells, with prominent cytoplasmic processes entrapping individual collagen fibers.

These findings contrast with those observed in normal capillaries, in which the dendritic nature of the pericytes and their relationship to the capillary wall have been clearly defined anatomically (59). Lymphatic capillaries, on the other hand, lack a prominent basal lamina and similarly lack dendritic pericytes (60). McNutt et al. (57) made the statement that "these features occasionally make it difficult to distinguish the small blood vessels in Kaposi's sarcoma from lymphatic channels." They further state, "the similarity between patch stage Kaposi's sarcoma vessels and lymphatics is also occasionally striking at the light microscopic level when the Kaposi's sarcoma vessels contain few erythrocytes and have an associated collection of small lymphocytes and plasma cells. The striking similarities in structure between Kaposi's sarcoma vessels and lymphatics have additional implications in that some cases of Kaposi's sarcoma appear to involve the lymphatic system. The high frequency of lymph node involvement by cutaneous Kaposi's sarcoma and the occasional primary lymph node Kaposi's sarcoma case can be interpreted to imply an origin of Kaposi's sarcoma in lymphatic vessels."

Having made these crucial observations, McNutt et al. then proceed to cite reports indicating that the distinction between the vessels in Kaposi's sarcoma and lymphatic endothelium has been clarified by the demonstration that the cells lining vessels in Kaposi's sarcoma and the spindle cells stain for factor VIII-related antigen (FVIIIRAg) and for alkaline phosphatase in a manner similar to that of blood vessel endothelium (61,62). As indicated below, our own observations and those reported by others, based on enzyme histochemical and immunohistochemical studies, are at variance with those cited by McNutt et al. and provide support for the contention that Kaposi's sarcoma is a proliferative disorder of lymphatic endothelium. We recognize nonetheless that the spindle cell areas may also comprise reactive fibroblasts, myofibroblasts, and histiocytes.

The personal observations of Dorfman (48), based on electron microscopic studies of biopsies from adult Africans and heterosexual men in the United States, are identical to those described by McNutt et al. in early lesions of Kaposi's sarcoma in homosexual men (57). These features included the presence of necrotic endothelial cells, fragmentation of basal lamina, and breaks in the continuity of the capillary endothelium (Figure 9), providing a mechanism for the extravasation of erythrocytes, presumed to enter the lymphatic system via abnormal lymphatic-venous anastomoses (42–44).

Ultrastructural studies have also been utilized in the search for viruses, suggested as etiologic agents in the induction of Kaposi's sarcoma, by a number of participants at the Kampala symposium. Evidence of an association between Kaposi's sarcoma and one or other viruses emerged some 10 years later, when Giraldo et al. (4) identified herpes-type virus particles in established tissue culture cell lines obtained from biopsy material from African patients. More recently, Walter et al. (63) claim to have identified a few "intranuclear herpes-type viral inclusions" in a Kaposi's sarcoma cell of the endothelial type, in biopsy material obtained from one of three African patients with typical nodular cutaneous tumors. They stated that their findings complemented previous reports of herpes-type viral particles in Kaposi's sarcoma cultured cell lines and suggest that, at least under certain conditions, Kaposi's sarcoma cells enter a virus-producing phase.

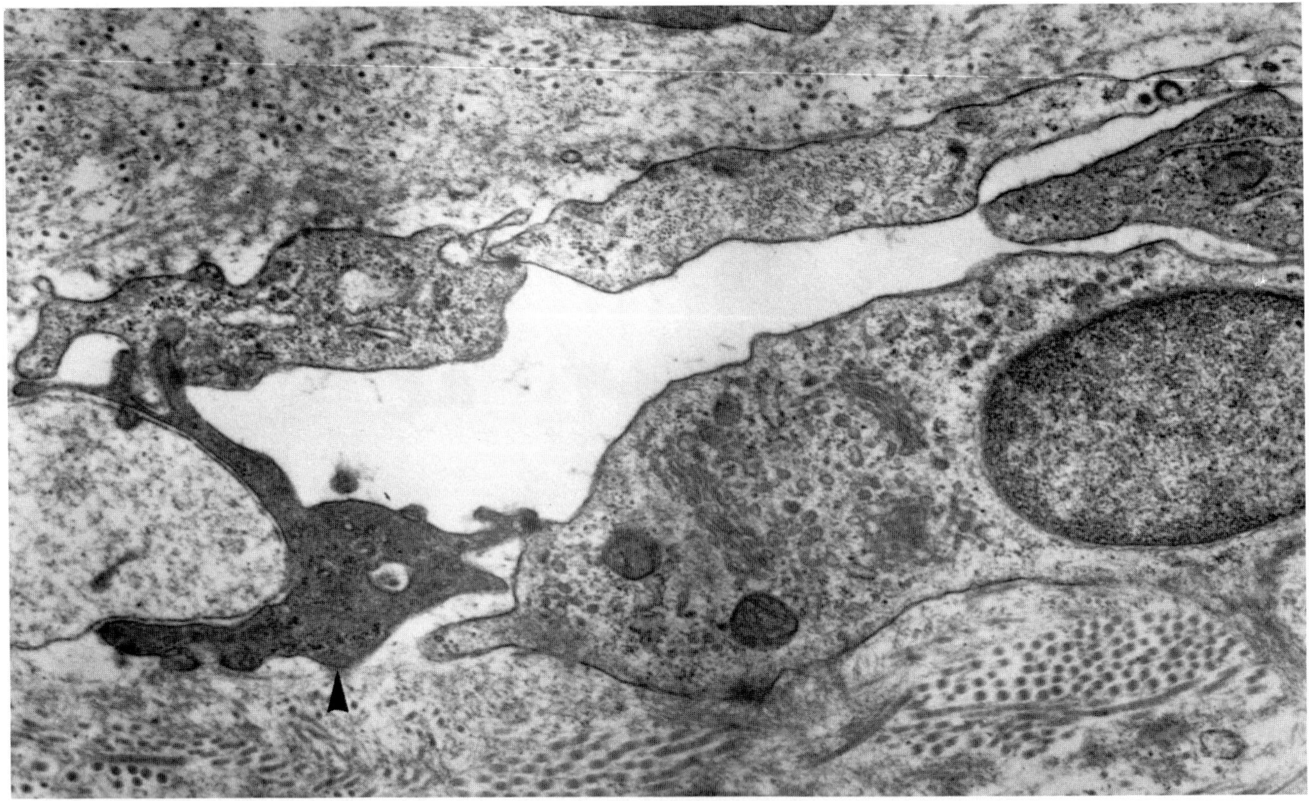

Figure 9 Cutaneous Kaposi's sarcoma in an elderly heterosexual man. A small capillary shows discontinuity of the endothelium, with fragmentation of the basal lamina and degenerative changes in the cytoplasm of one shrunken endothelial cell (arrow). (Uranyl acetate and lead citrate stain, ×15,000) (Reprinted with permission from W. B. Saunders Company. Dorfman RF. Kaposi's sarcoma revisited. Hum Pathol 1984; 15:1013–7.)

ENZYME HISTOCHEMICAL STUDIES

The majority of reported histochemical studies have applied enzyme histochemical methods to the investigation of Kaposi's sarcoma. A review of the literature on the reported findings of various investigators discloses an extraordinary difference of opinion relating to the activity of a wide variety of enzymes in the spindle cells of Kaposi's sarcoma. The discrepancies in findings from one report to another could well be accounted for by technical differences and/or by the different substrates utilized by these investigators. The earliest reports were those of Kopf in 1957 (64) and Pepler in 1959 (37). Kopf studied alkaline phosphatase, an ezyme known to show strong activity in the endothelial cells of blood vascular capillaries. He reported mild alkaline phosphatase activity in the early stage, zero to mild activity in the advanced papular phase, and strong positivity in the sarcomatous stage. In contrast, Pepler failed to identify any alkaline phosphatase in the spindle cells but reported the expression of nonspecific esterase and strong pseudocholinesterase activity in the spindle cells. According to Pepler, the endothelial cells lining capillaries showed only alkaline phosphatase activity.

Becker (17) and Dorfman (43) reported at the Kampala symposium that we were similarly unable to identify evidence of alkaline phosphatase activity in the spindle cells; nor were we able to confirm Pepler's finding of pseudocholinesterase activity. The latter observation, in conjunction with Pepler's electron microscopic studies, was taken as evidence of origin of the spindle cells from Schwann cells. Pepler's findings have not been confirmed by others, and as indicated previously, the lamellated membranous structures described by Pepler and Theron (51) and interpreted by them as schwannian myelin sheath are considered to represent residual bodies of lysosomes.

Becker (17) reported that the endothelial cells lining vessels showed only alkaline phosphatase activity whereas the spindle cells of Kaposi's sarcoma expressed acid phosphatase, some eserine resistant esterase, adenosine triphosphatase, and mild acid pyrophosphatase acitvity. Despite his inability to confirm the findings of Pepler, Becker nonetheless maintained that the cellular source of Kaposi's sarcoma was likely to be the perivascular Schwann cell.

Dorfman (43) presented the results of a study of hydrolytic enzyme activity in Kaposi's sarcoma at the Kampala symposium.

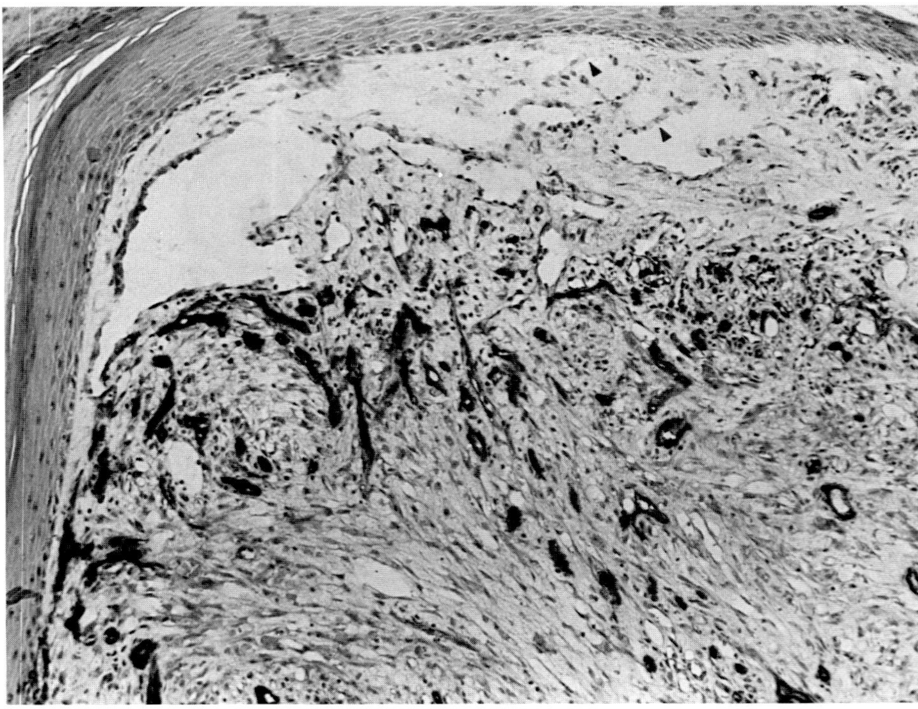

Figure 10 Cutaneous Kaposi's sarcoma in a heterosexual adult African. Alkaline phosphatase activity is evident in the endothelial cells lining capillaries in the middermis but spindle cells in the lower dermis and endothelium lining dilated lymphatics in the upper dermis (small arrows) show no activity of this enzyme. (Calcium-cobalt method; nuclear fast red counterstain, ×120) (Reprinted with permission from S. Karger A.G., Basel. Dorfman RF. Kaposi's sarcoma; the contribution of enzyme histochemistry to the identification of cell types. Acta Union Int Contre Cancer 1962; 18:464–76.)

Strong alkaline phosphatase activity was noted in the endothelium of blood vascular capillaries in the dermis (Figure 10), and zero to mildly positive acid phosphatase and nonspecific esterase activity was observed in these cells. In contrast, the endothelial cells lining normal lymphatics and lymphangiomatous spaces showed no expression of alkaline phosphatase (Figure 11) and zero to 1+ nonspecific esterase activity. Expression of cholinesterase was not

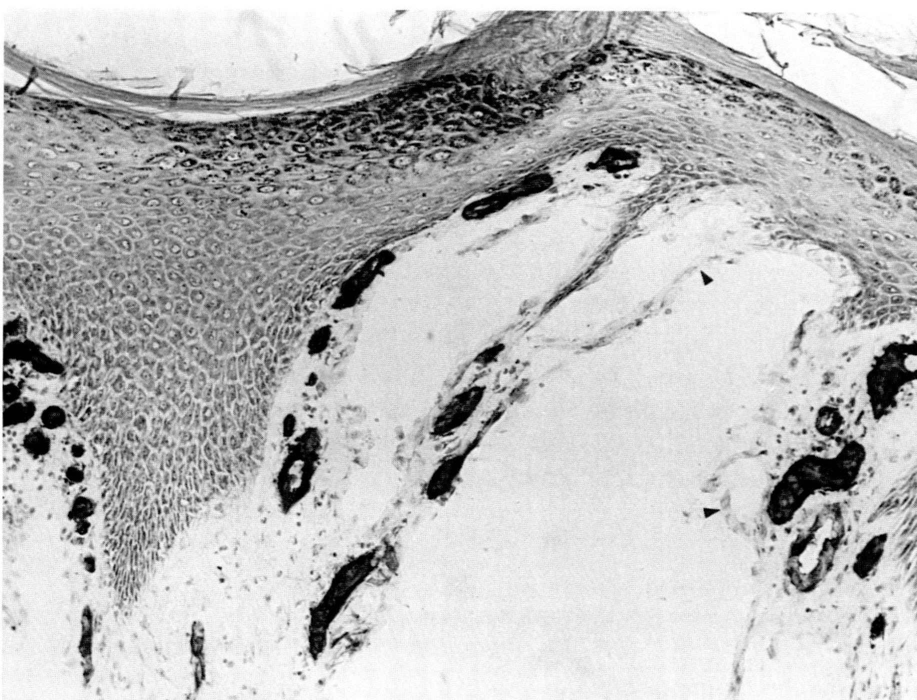

Figure 11 Cutaneous lymphangioma. Alkaline phosphatase activity is localized in endothelium of blood capillaries, but not in endothelium lining dilated lymphatic spaces (small arrows). (Calcium cobalt method; nuclear fast red counterstain, ×120) (Reprinted with permission from S. Karger A.G., Basel. Dorfman RF. Kaposi's sarcoma; the contribution of enzyme histochemistry to the identification of cell types. Acta Union Int Contre Cancer 1962; 18:464–76.)

identified in any of the cellular elements comprising Kaposi's sarcoma, other than nerve fibers that might be encompassed in or infiltrated by the tumor. The *absence* of alkaline phosphatase activity in the spindle cells of Kaposi's sarcoma in this study (Figure 10) was considered to be strong evidence against their origin from blood vessel endothelium or from fibroblasts. The inability to demonstrate cholinesterase activity was taken as evidence against their neural origin. The presence of only minimal nonspecific esterase and acid phosphatase activity in some spindle cells was considered insufficient evidence of their derivation from the reticuloendothelial system. It was postulated by Dorfman that multicentric neoformation of lymphatics is a primary process in the histogenesis of Kaposi's sarcoma and that the predominant localization corresponds to the normal distribution of lymphatics.

In 1964, Hashimoto and Lever (52) reported the results of their histochemical studies on Kaposi's sarcoma and concluded that the tumor was composed mainly of two types of cells, endothelial cells and phagocytic fibroblasts. They reported the presence of lysosomes in both endothelial cells and fibroblasts by means of electron microscopy and histochemical staining and further indicated that stains for nonspecific alkaline phosphatase showed various stages of maturation from immature to well-formed vascular elements. They further stated that an intense reaction of acid phosphatase and a moderate to strong reaction of β-glucuronidase in the granules of the perivascular tumor cells indicated that these cells are capable of phagocytosis and that their granules represent lysosomes seen by electron microscopy.

More recently, Beckstead and Wood (45) reported their findings in biopsy specimens from 40 patients with Kaposi's sarcoma, utilizing enzyme histochemistry and immunohistochemistry (Figures 12 through 15). They concluded that the phenotype of neoplastic cells in Kaposi's sarcoma closely resembled that of lymphatic endothelium but not of blood vessel endothelium, as discussed in the following section.

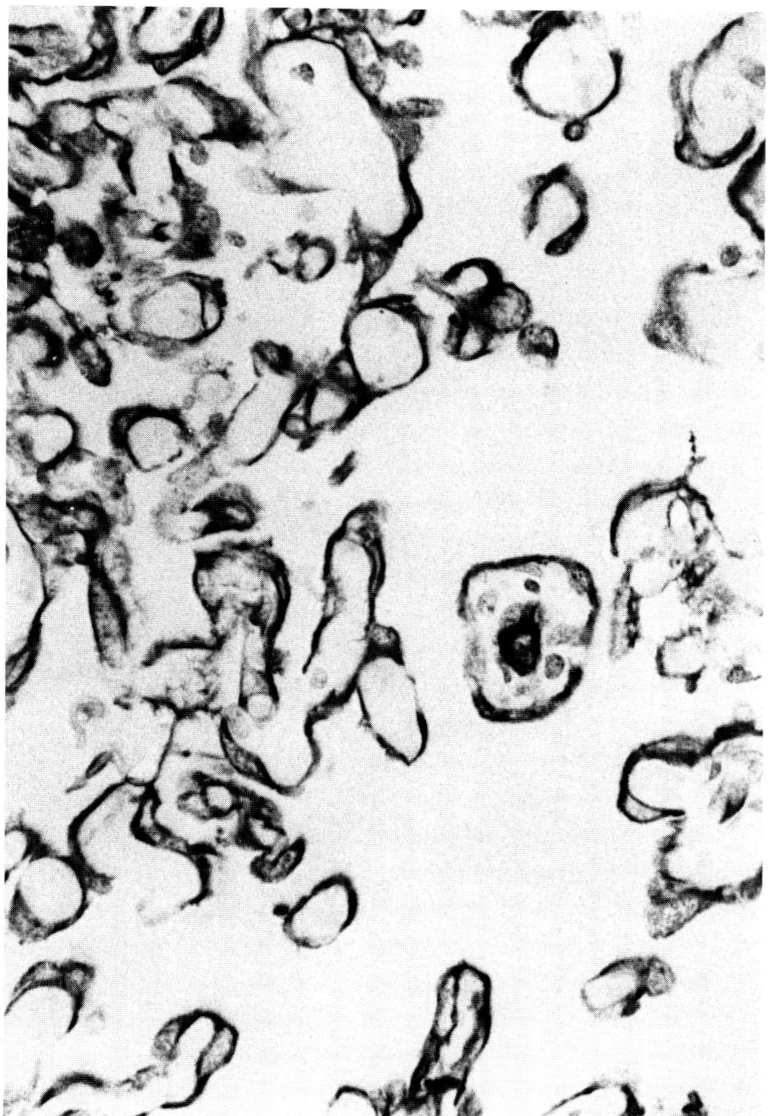

Figure 12 Kaposi's sarcoma in the skin. The endothelial cells lining the irregular vascular spaces are labeled by the endothelial marker, *Ulex europeaus*. (Plastic section counterstained with neutral red, ×400)

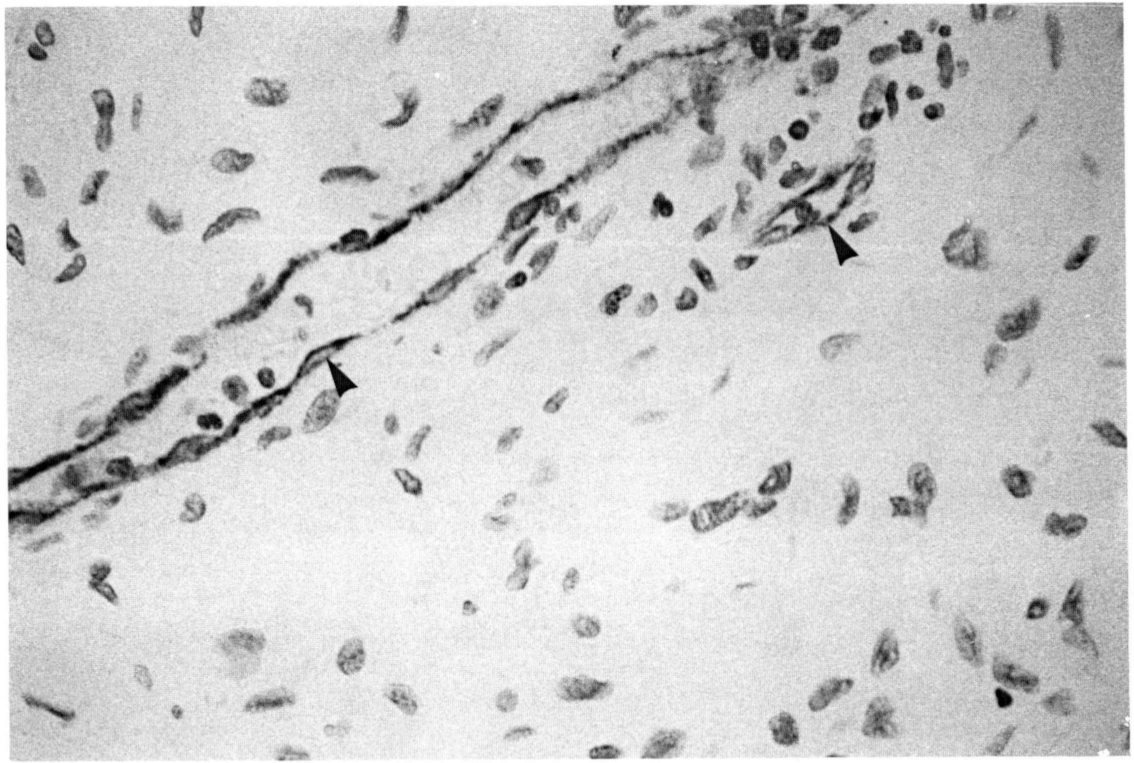

Figure 13 Kaposi's sarcoma in the skin. The spindle cells show no labeling with FVIIIRAg (same lesion as Figure 12), but scattered blood vessels within the lesion are well stained (arrows). (Plastic section counterstained with neutral red, ×400)

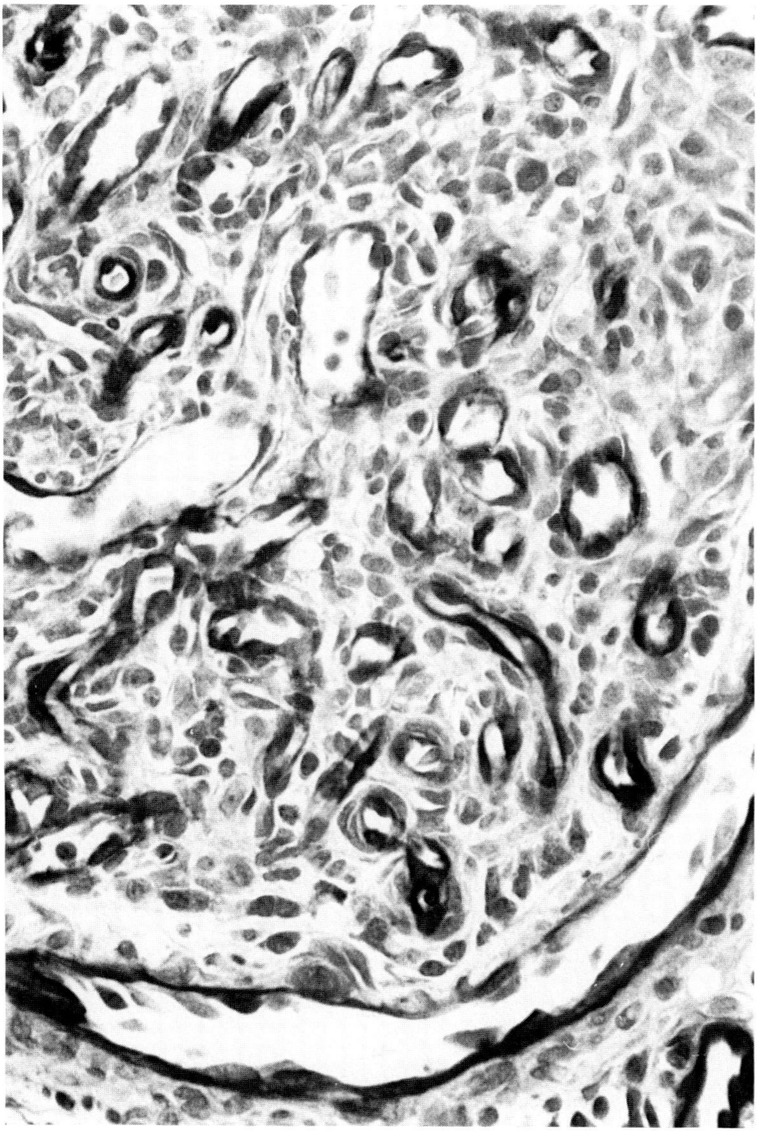

Figure 14 Kaposi's sarcoma in a lymph node. The numerous normal blood vessels in the lesion shown in Figure 7 are demonstrated well with the alkaline phosphatase reaction, which stains normal capillaries and venules dark blue and leaves the abnormal cells unstained. (Plastic section counterstained with neutral red, ×400)

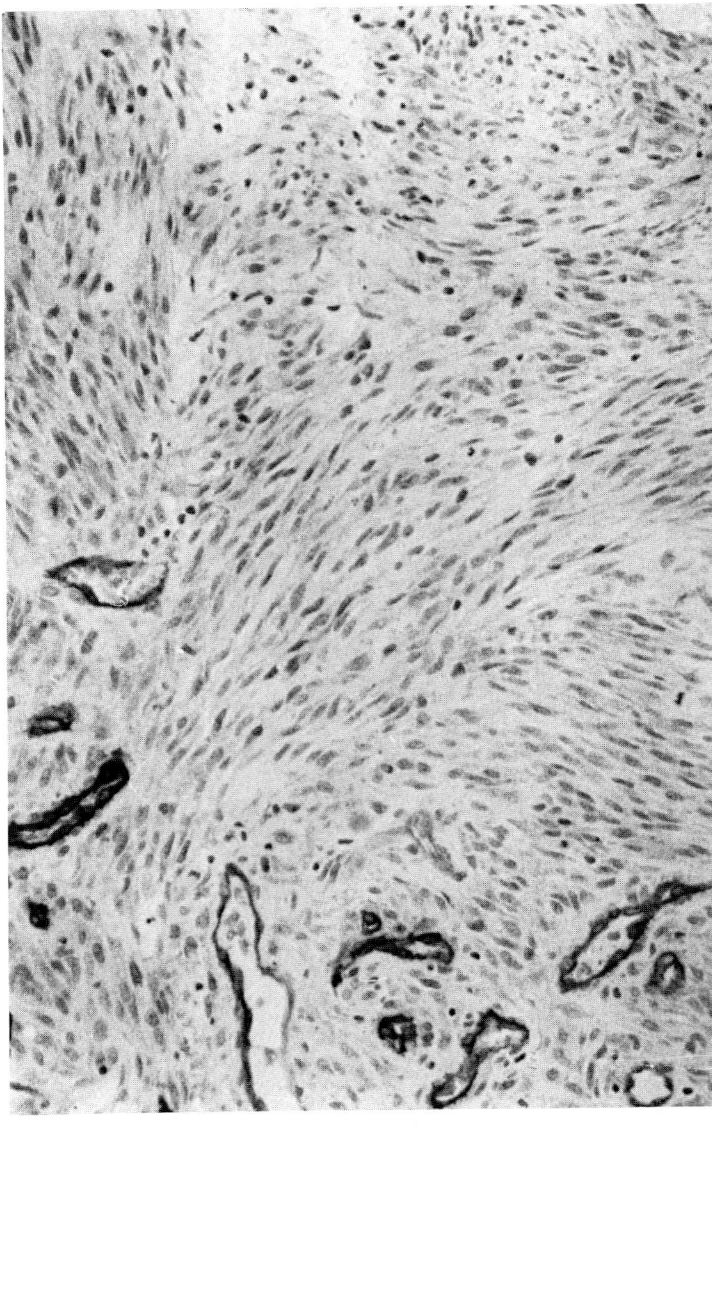

Figure 15 Kaposi's sarcoma in a lymph node. The dark alkaline phosphatase reaction demonstrates the residual normal vessels, which are gradually replaced by the proliferating abnormal spindle cells. (Plastic section counterstained with neutral red, ×160)

IMMUNOHISTOCHEMISTRY

The advent of monoclonal antibodies (MoAb) (2) has provided investigators with an extraordinary opportunity to define the nature of cells in health and disease and, in many instances, to distinguish hyperplasia from neoplasia. Although many of these techniques require fresh-frozen material, a number of MoAb can be applied to fixed tissues embedded in paraffin or plastic, utilizing a variety of immunoperoxidase methods. Initally described by Sternberger (65), the peroxidase-antiperoxidase method (PAP) has been widely used to identify antigens as immunohistologic markers for a variety of cell types. In 1981, Guarda et al. (61) and Nadji et al. (62), employing similar techniques, independently reported the presence of factor VIII-related antigen (FVIIIRAg) in the endothelial cells lining vascular channels and blood-filled clefts, in addition to the spindle cells of Kaposi's sarcoma. Since FVIIIRAg is apparently elaborated mainly by endothelial cells, mast cells, platelets, and megakaryocytes, these investigators concluded that the immunologic reaction for this factor in the spindle cells of Kaposi's sarcoma strongly supported a vascular endothelial derivation. They emphasized that lymphatic endothelium failed to elaborate FVIIIRAg.

These findings were received with great interest and enthusiasm by the scientific community and seemed finally to have resolved the controversy over the nature of the spindle cells. Unfortunately, subsequent studies by several independent workers utilizing polyclonal and monoclonal antibodies, in addition to heteroantisera, have consistently failed to identify FVIIIRAg staining of the spindle cells in Kaposi's sarcoma (11,45,66,67). Moreover, controversy has been renewed by Svanholm et al. (68), who reported positive cytoplasmic staining for FVIIIRAg in lymphatic vessels.

These conflicting results have raised the issue of variation in antibody specificity and sensitivity and of differences in methodology. Millard and Heryet (66), who reported no labeling of the tumor spindle cells for FVIIIRAg, utilizing two commercially available polyclonal antibodies and three monoclonal antibodies, have discussed these discrepancies indicating that explanations for these differing observations have included variation of antigen synthesis, the size of the putative cell, and the possible suppression of antigen synthesis by tumor or dedifferentiation of the endothelial cell. In reported studies describing widespread labeling for FVIIIRAg in frozen sections of tumor, they suggest that, given the considerable vascular component of Kaposi's sarcoma, it is obviously possible that leakage of FVIIIRAg could occur in frozen tissues and so contribute to the widespread labeling of spindle cells reported. They emphasize that the use of formalin-fixed tissue should overcome these criticisms. The divergent observations could also be explained by the absence of a definition of what is accepted as positive labeling. This becomes clear after careful study of the illustrations in a number of reports.

The problem of nonspecific background staining for FVIIIRAg was addressed by Beckstead et al. (45). They failed to identify a consistent pattern related to the source of antibody. Moreover, they observed no significant differences in their reactions using four different antibodies. They also drew attention to reports of spurious staining in paraffin sections (false-negative as well as false-positive results) (69) particularly relating to FVIIIRAg (70). Utilizing a combination of enzyme histochemistry and immunohistochemistry, they have applied seven markers to characterize the endothelial cells and spindle cells of Kaposi's sarcoma in plastic and frozen sections (Figures 12 through 15). These markers include three types of antigens (FVIIIRAg, HLA-DR/Ia, and macrophage-endothelial antigens), three enzymes (5′-nucleotidase, ATPase, and alkaline phosphatase) and lectin binding (*Ulex europaeus* I). They applied these markers to normal skin and lymph node and to biopsy specimens from 40 patients with Kaposi's sarcoma. Normal blood vessel endothelium showed reactivity for all seven markers, but normal lymphatic endothelium and most of the spindle cells were negative for all markers except 5′-nucleotidase and *U. europaeus* lectin (Figure 12). Their study demonstrated that the phenotype of the abnormal proliferating cell in

Kaposi's sarcoma differed significantly from that of nonneoplastic blood vessel endothelium. The phenotype demonstrated (FVIIIRAg-negative [Figure 13], HLA-DR/Ia-negative, Mo/E-negative, UEA-positive, ATP-negative, Alkø-negative [Figure 15], 5′-nucleotidase-positive) closely resembles the phenotype of normal lymphatic endothelium. They further demonstrated that plastic sections completely eliminate any localization problems. Although it is possible that the plastic technique may be insensitive to extremely small amounts of FVIIIRAg detectable by other techniques, it is unlikely that significant amounts of FVIIIRAg were undetectable in frozen sections, which they also utilized. They concluded, therefore, that the neoplastic cells in 40 cases of Kaposi's sarcoma closely resembled the phenotype of normal lymphatic endothelium, but not of blood vessel endothelium. Thus, their studies suggested that the cellular origin of Kaposi's sarcoma is the lymphatic endothelial cell, in concordance with Dorfman's hypothesis (43), proposed some 25 years ago. The predilection for lymph nodes, often without skin lesions, reported in African children (38,71) and more recently in homosexual men (72) and in children with AIDS (38,73) appears to provide strong support for this hypothesis.

Recognizing that immunohistochemical staining for FVIIIRAg in Kaposi's sarcoma led to conflicting results and that this antigen clearly was not a reliable and reproducible immunohistochemical marker for the spindle cell component of Kaposi's sarcoma, Rutgers et al. (74) utilized monoclonal antibodies that detect three distinctive vascular endothelial cell-associated antigens, E92, OKM5, and HCL. At the outset they also noted absent, weak, or focal and variable expression of FVIIIRAg, consistent with the observations of other investigators. In contrast, they reported strong reactivity of the spindle cell component in each of 19 lesions, with OKM5 and with anti-E92 and weak reactivity with anti-HCL. A subpopulation of spindle cells also expressed HLA-DR (Ia) antigen. They also indicated that prior studies with multiple samples from a diverse group of human tissues have failed to disclose any obvious expression of these antigens by lymphatic endothelium. The cells lining dermal lymphatics and nodal lymphatic sinuses conspicuously lack E92, OKM5, and HCL. Their observation that the spindle cells of Kaposi's sarcoma consistently express HLA-DR antigens, as does normal vascular endothelium, contrasts with our reported results. They recognized, nonetheless, that this discrepancy could be related to technique or choice of monoclonal anti-HLA-DR, but they concluded that their observations provided "the strongest and most compelling evidence thus far for the vascular endothelial cell origin of the spindled cell component of Kaposi's sarcoma." In the light of the conflicting results with FVIIIRAg, it remains for other workers to confirm the findings of Rutgers et al. It may also be pertinent to point out that recent immunohistochemical studies have identified phenotypic subsets of endothelial cells that correlate with specific morphological subtypes (75). These include (1) arterioles, capillaries, and venules; (2) high endothelial venules and hepatic sinusoidal lining cells; (3) lymphatics and glomerular capillaries; (4) splenic sinusoidal lining cells; and (5) umbilical cord endothelial cells. Moreover, some of these endothelial cells share functional and phenotypic properties with cells of the monocyte-macrophage lineage.

In yet another immunohistochemical approach to the question of histogenesis, Bendelac et al. (76) and Kramer et al. (77) have used frozen section techniques to identify the presence of basement membrane proteins, collagen type IV, and laminin. This approach was based on the studies by Barsky et al. (78), the results of which suggested that lymphatic capillaries could be distinguished from blood vascular capillaries by the absence of basal lamina proteins. These investigators identified basement membrane proteins in Kaposi's sarcoma and concluded that this tumor must therefore be of blood vascular origin. Two criticisms, one minor and one major, may be raised. The contribution of normal reactive vessels is not considered, but more importantly the basic premise is less clear-cut than indicated in these papers. Barsky et al. clearly state that the larger lymphatic channels have well-defined basal lamina. On the other hand, they cite electron microscopic studies by Leak (60) that reveal that lymphatic capillaries have a poorly formed and discontinuous basal lamina rather than a complete absence of this structure. This would suggest that the presence or absence of basement membrane proteins may not provide clear-cut distinctions between cells of vascular and lymphatic origin. Furthermore, the presence of large amounts of basal lamina proteins in these lesions is certainly at odds with the electron microscopic observations of Dorfman (56) and of McNutt (57). In a more recent study, Jones et al. (79) found weak staining for laminin in Kaposi's lesions and in dermal lymphatics, findings more in keeping with ultrastructural observations. They also utilized two new monoclonal antibodies reactive with endothelial cells, as well as the lectin UEA and FVIIIRAg. Based on the application of these techniques to 30 biopsies, they strongly favored a lymphatic origin for Kaposi's sarcoma.

OTHER EXPERIMENTAL METHODS

Tissue Culture

As with many other tumors, the objectives of tissue culture are, first, to establish cell lines in continuous culture, with the expectation that these will show recognizable cellular differentiation; and second, hope that such cell lines may elaborate one or more viruses that would prove to represent the etiologic agent. At the Kampala symposium, Spence (80) gave a preliminary report dealing with the isolation and growth in tissue culture of a strain of cells said to derive from a biopsy of a skin nodule of Kaposi's sarcoma in an African patient. These cells were said to be "epithelioid in character and to resemble those derived from malignant epidermoid carcinomas." From this description it is unlikely that the cell lines represented the spindle cell of Kaposi's sarcoma, and no subsequent reports were forthcoming from this investigator.

Davison, Karasek, and Bensch (81,82) have described a procedure for isolation and in vitro cultivation of endothelial cells. Moreover, they have succeeded in modulating the growth of these cells by the inclusion of varying amounts of cyclic AMP in the culture medium. Their criteria for establishing the endothelial origin of isolated cells included the characteristic cellular morphology of the growth pattern at the light microscopic level; ultrastructural characteristics, including the presence of Weibel-Palade bodies, determined by electron microscopy, and the presence of factor VIII-associated protein by indirect immunofluorescence. Karasek (83) has also indicated that he is similarly able to modulate factor VIII expression in endothelial cells by varying cAMP levels and that the more spindled cells show weaker reactivity for FVIIIRAg. By extrapolation, these observations may account for some of the discrepancies reported in the literature regarding the immunoreactivity of spindle cells of Kaposi's sarcoma to FVIIIRAg. Such observations also suggest that it may be important to manipulate Kaposi's sarcoma cells in culture to determine whether these cells can be induced to change their phenotype.

Giraldo and his associates (4) have utilized tissue culture as a means of identifying virus particles by electron microscopy and have reported the presence of both herpesvirus particles and particles resembling cytomegalovirus. These investigators succeeded in establishing 51 cell lines in continuous culture from 40 cases of Kaposi's sarcoma, and some have been continuously propagated for a number of years. Of these cell lines, 25 were derived from tumor nodules, 16 from lymph nodes draining sites of nodules of Kaposi's sarcoma, and 10 from normal skin. They reported that long-term cultures had irregular growth patterns of either fibroblastoid cells or cells with an epithelioid pattern and that the cells did not exhibit contact inhibition. Considerable pleomorphism was noted in the cultures, and electron microscopy revealed herpesvirus particles in 5 of 8 lines examined. They indicated that in another line, in which the cells were more epithelioid in type (the herpesvirus lines were fibroblastoid or had undergone a change to a cell that seemed to have the characteristics of a macrophage), cytomegalovirus was identified. Preliminary immunologic studies indicated antigens in common with Epstein-Barr virus but of low titer (5). All the patients with Kaposi's sarcoma in this study originated from Uganda or Zaire.

Giraldo et al. also claimed to have detected CMV-related antigens in neoplastic cells in tissue culture and in biopsy specimens (3), and Fenoglio et al. (84), utilizing DNA hybridization studies, have demonstrated CMV DNA within the neoplastic cells of Kaposi's sarcoma. On the other hand, Cerimele et al. (85) reported their failure to demonstrate early and late antigens of cytomegalovirus in tissue cultures from Kaposi's sarcoma patients utilizing immunoperoxidase antibody techniques. These observations on virologic studies are covered in greater detail elsewhere in this publication.

Experimental Reproduction of the Disease

In his elegant and comprehensive presentation at the Kampala symposium, Oettlé (86) indicated that the induction of malignant angiomatous tumors in laboratory animals had been achieved with a number of carcinogenic agents. None of these, however, had induced lesions resembling Kaposi's sarcoma. He also discussed the possibility that Kaposi's sarcoma may be caused by an infectious agent attacking the entire vascular and perivascular system, producing the early stages of the lesion, assuming neoplastic properties in the late stages or under particular conditions. He emphasized that the large number of failures to prove transmission by inoculation into humans and into animals remained an obstacle to this hypothesis. Oettlé and Kaminer (87) attempted to inoculate fresh tissue from a case of Kaposi's sarcoma into 10 mice without success. Becker and Thatcher (88) established tissue cultures from a case of Kaposi's sarcoma for 6 days and apparently obtained successful implantation into the skin of the donor; however, tissue implanted into rabbits failed to grow and successful subculture was not proven.

Is Kaposi's Sarcoma a Malignant Tumor?

As indicated recently by Lo and Liotta (89), the varied histopathology of Kaposi's sarcoma has engendered controversy concerning its histogenesis and neoplastic nature. Some investigators have proposed that it is a sarcoma derived from primitive mesenchymal cells; however, others consider this lesion a benign proliferative disorder. Costa and Rabson (90) suggest that the multiple nodules are autochthonous rather than metastatic. Lo and Liotta approached this controversy by searching for transforming gene(s) associated with Kaposi's sarcoma occurring in patients with AIDS. Their findings appear to provide a powerful argument for the neoplastic nature of Kaposi's sarcoma. They reported that DNA obtained from Kaposi's sarcoma tissue successfully transformed phenotypically normal NIH/3T3 cells: when injected into nude mice the transfected lines produced vascular tumors, which they considered histopathologically similar to Kaposi's sarcoma. Thus Lo and Liotta suggested that DNA from Kaposi's sarcoma may contain one or more distinct transforming genes.

An additional alternative to consider is the concept of multiclonal tumors analogous to the lymphomas described by Cleary and associates (91,92) in heart transplant recipients. They reported different clones of neoplastic lymphoid cells, each expressing different immunoglobulin gene rearrangements. Such multiclonal lymphomas may well be induced by a virus, such as the Epstein-Barr virus, in the setting of immunodeficiency secondary to treatment of transplant recipients with steroids and cyclosporin A. The multicentric distribution of lesions of Kaposi's sarcoma in AIDS could be explained on an analogous basis; in this case the offending virus may be cytomegalovirus and the immunodeficiency induced by human immunodeficiency virus (HIV).

SUMMARY

Moritz Kaposi's description in 1872 of the tumor that bears his name and that he termed idiopathic multiple pigmented sarcoma of the skin clearly provides evidence that he considered this to be malignant. He stated, "according to the experience available, the disease must be considered from the outset not only incurable, but also lethal." Nonetheless, the astonishing variety of descriptive terms utilized by numerous authors during the ensuing 85 years (prior to the publication of Bluefarb's book in 1957) reflects the varying concepts of the nature of this disease and of its histogenesis. To this day the controversy persists. Initial concepts were based on morphological observations at the light microscopic level, correlated to some extent with clinical behavior and course of the disease. Enzyme histochemical studies produced conflicting results and hypotheses. Electron microscopy identified an apparent mixture of component cells, without demonstrating specific or diagnostic ultrastructural features. Although the establishment of continuous cell lines in tissue culture has similarly failed to provide evidence of cellular differentiation, such methods have been useful in the identification of viral particles considered to play a role in the causation of Kaposi's sarcoma. With the advent of monoclonal antibodies it was hoped that their application to the study of this tumor would finally provide the answer to the riddle of this "mysterious" sarcoma; however, a number of conflicting reports have appeared in the literature, particularly in regard to factor VIII-related antigen, reported by some workers to provide evidence of the origin of Kaposi's sarcoma from vascular endothelial cells, observations denied by others. In view of the conflicting results with FVIIIRAg it remains for other workers to confirm and extend these findings as additional antibodies specific for various endothelial subsets become available.

The weight of evidence based on light microscopic and morbid anatomic observations, supported by the distribution of lesions in the skin, submucosa of the gastrointestinal tract, and lymph nodes (often without skin lesions); the absence of lesions in organs devoid of lymphatics, that is, the brain and eyeball; and the results of electron microscopic, enzyme histochemical, and immunohistochemical studies performed by the authors and by others seem to favor derivation of the neoplastic spindle cell of Kaposi's sarcoma from lymphatic endothelium. We recognize, nonetheless, that reactive elements, such as fibroblasts, myofibroblasts, and histiocytes, may also be involved in the proliferative process.

ACKNOWLEDGMENTS

Supported in part by grants CA-05838, CA-34233, CA-33119, and CA-2155 from the National Institutes of Health, by the University of California Task Force on AIDS, and by grants CA-24264-109 from the United States Public Health Service.

REFERENCES

1. Kaposi M, Idiopathisches multiples pigment-sarkom der haut. Arch Dermatol Syph 1872; 4:265–73. (English translation, CA 1982; 32:342–7.
2. Kohler H, Milstein C. Continuous cultures of fused cells secreting antibody of predefined specificity. Nature 1975; 256:495–7.
3. Giraldo G, Beth E. The involvement of cytomegalovirus in acquired immune deficiency syndrome and Kaposi's sarcoma. Prog Allergy 1986; 37:319–31.
4. Giraldo G, Beth E, Haguenau F. Herpes-type virus particles in tissue culture of Kaposi's sarcoma from different geographic regions. JNCI 1972; 49:1509–26.
5. Giraldo G, Beth E, Kourilsky FM, Henle W, Mike V, Huraux JM, Anderson HK, Garbi MR, Kyalwazi SK, Puissan TA. Antibody patterns to herpes viruses in Kaposi's sarcoma: serological association of European Kaposi's sarcoma with cytomegalovirus. Int J Cancer 1975; 15:839–48.
6. Gallo RC, Salahuddin SZ, Popovic M, et al. Frequent detection of cytopathic retroviruses (HTLV-III) from patients with AIDS and at risk for AIDS. Science 1984; 224:500–3.
7. Barré-Sinoussi F, Cherman JC, Ray F, et al. Isolation of a T-lymphotrophic retrovirus from a patient at risk for acquired immune deficiency syndrome (AIDS). Science 1983; 220:868–71.
8. Goudsmit J, deWolf F, Paul D, et al. Expression of human immunodeficiency virus antigen (HIV-Ag) in serum and cerebrospinal fluid during acute and chronic infection. Lancet 1986; 2:177–9.
9. Myers BD, Kessler E, Levi J, et al. Kaposi's sarcoma in kidney transplant recipients. Arch Intern Med 1974; 133:307–11.
10. Penn I. Kaposi's sarcoma in organ transplant recipients: report of 20 cases. Transplantation 1979; 27:8–11.

11. Akhtar M, Bunuan H, Ali MA, Godwin JT. Kaposi's sarcoma in renal transplant recipients. Ultrastructural and immunoperoxidase study of four cases. Cancer 1984; 53:258–66.
12. Ziegler JL, Templeton AC, Vogel CL, Kaposi's sarcoma: a comparison of classical, endemic, and epidemic forms. Semin Oncol 1984; 11:47–52.
13. Volberding PA. Kaposi's sarcoma and the acquired immunodeficiency syndrome. Med Clin North Am 1986; 70:665–75.
14. Symposium on Kaposi's sarcoma. Acta Union Int Contre Cancer 1962; 18:322–511.
15. Roulet FC. Comments on the possible histogenesis of the cellular components of the so-called "haemangiosarcoma Kaposi." Acta Union Int Contre Cancer 1962; 18:460–4.
16. Murray JL, Lothe F. The histopathology of Kaposi's sarcoma. Acta Union Int Contre Cancer 1962; 18:413–28.
17. Becker BJP. The histogenesis of Kaposi's sarcoma. Acta Union Int Contre Cancer 1962; 18:477–86.
18. Choisser RM, Ramsay EM. Angio-reticuloendothelioma of the heart (Kaposi disease). Am J Pathol 1939; 15:155–78.
19. Dorffel J. Histogenesis of multiple idiopathic hemorrhagic sarcoma. Arch Dermatol Syph 1932; 26:608–34.
20. Tedeschi CG, Folsom HF, Carnicelli TJ. Visceral Kaposi disease. Arch Pathol 1947; 43:335–57.
21. McCarthy WD, Pack GT. Malignant blood vessel tumors. Surg Gynecol Obstet 1950; 91:465–82.
22. Osborne ED, Jordan JW, Hoak FC, Pschierer FJ. Nitrogen mustard therapy in cutaneous blastomatous disease. JAMA 1947; 135:1123–8.
23. Pautrier LM, Diss A. Kaposi sarcoma is not a genuine sarcoma but a neurovascular dysgenesis. Br J Dermatol 1929; 41:93–105.
24. Ewing J. *Neoplastic Disease*. Philadelphia, WB Saunders, 1940.
25. McKee GM, Cipollaro AC. Idiopathic multiple hemorrhagic sarcoma (Kaposi). Am J Cancer 1936; 26:1–27.
26. Aegerter EE, Peale AR. Kaposi sarcoma—a critical survey. Arch Pathol (Chicago) 1942; 34:413–22.
27. Fraser JF. Kaposi sarcoma. Arch Dermatol Syph 1933; 28:143–4.
28. Sachs W, Azulay RD, Convit J. Multiple idiopathic hemorrhagic sarcoma of Kaposi—a histopathological study. J Invest Dermatol 1947; 8:317–26.

29. Philippson L. Über das sarcoma idiopathicum cutis Kaposi; Ein beitrag zur sarcomlehre. Arch Pathol Anat 1902; 167:58–87.
30. Schwimmer EL. Sarcoma, idiopathische hautsarkom multiplex cutis (abstract). Monatschr Prakt Dermatol 1899; 9:90.
31. Symmers D. Kaposi's disease. Arch Pathol 1941; 32:764–86.
32. Sternberg C. Uber das sarcoma multiplex hemorrhagicum (Kaposi). Arch Dermatol Syph 1912; 111:331–40.
33. Bernhardt R. Sarcomata idiopathica multiplica pigmentosa cutis (Kaposi). Arch Dermatol Syph 1899; 49:207–26.
34. Halle A. Ein Beitrag zur Kenntnis des Sarcoma idiopathicum multiplex hemorrhagicum (Kaposi). Arch Dermatol Syph 1904; 72:373–406.
35. Hamdi H, Resat H. Sur l'histologie de la sarcomatose de Kaposi (Acro-périthéliomatosa idiopathicum multiplex cavernosum lymphangiectoides cutaneum). Anal Anat Pathol 1932; 9:593–6.
36. Kusnezow WN. Case of sarcoma multiplex idiopathicum (Kaposi) with fatal outcome. Urol Cutan Rev 1933; 37:230–4.
37. Pepler WJ. The origin of Kaposi hemangiosarcoma, a histochemical study. J Pathol Bacteriol 1959; 78:553–7.
38. Dorfman RF. Kaposi's sarcoma: with special reference to its manifestations in infants and children and to the concepts of Arthur Purdy Stout. Am J Surg Pathol 1986; 10 (Suppl 1):68–77.
39. Stout AP. Kaposi's sarcoma. In: Tumors of the Soft Tissues (Atlas of Tumor Pathology, Sec. 2, Fac. 5), Washington D.C.; Armed Forces Institute of Pathology, 1953; 99:106.
40. Lothe F, Murray JL. Kaposi's sarcoma. Autopsy findings in the African. Acta Union Int Contre Cancer 1962; 18:116–39.
41. Yoffey JM, Courtice FC. *Lymphatics, Lymph and Lymphoid Tissue*, 2d ed. London, Edward Arnold, 1956.
42. Palmer PES. The radiological changes of Kaposi's sarcoma. Acta Union Int Contre Cancer 1962; 18:87–99.
43. Dorfman RF. Kaposi's sarcoma. The contribution of enzyme histochemistry to the identification of cell types. Acta Union Int Contre Cancer 1962; 18:151–63.
44. Dictor M. Kaposi's sarcoma. Origin and significance of lymphaticovenous connections. Virchows Arch (Pathol Anat) 1986; 409:23–35.
45. Beckstead JH, Wood GS, Fletcher V. Evidence for the origin of

Kaposi's sarcoma from lymphatic endothelium. Am J Pathol 1985; 119:294–300.
46. Camain R, Quenum A. Histopathology and histogenesis of Kaposi's disease. Acta Union Int Contre Cancer 1962; 18:140–6.
47. Lee FD. A comparative study of Kaposi's sarcoma and granuloma pyogenicum in Uganda. J Clin Pathol 1968; 21:119–28.
48. Dorfman RF. Kaposi's sarcoma revisited. Hum Pathol 1984; 15: 1013–7.
49. Templeton AC. Kaposi's sarcoma. In: Andrade R, Gumport SL, Popkin CL, et al, eds. Cancer of the Skin: Biology, Diagnosis and Management, Philadelphia, WB Saunders, 1976:1183–1225.
50. Bluefarb S. Kaposi's Sarcoma (Multiple Idiopathic Hemorrhagic Sarcoma). Springfield, Illinois, Charles C. Thomas, 1957.
51. Pepler WJ, Theron JJ. An electron-microscope study of Kaposi's haemangiosarcoma. J Pathol Bacteriol 1962; 83:521–5.
52. Hashimoto K, Lever WF. Kaposi's sarcoma: histochemical and electron microscopic studies. J Invest Dermatol 1964; 43:539–49.
53. Niemi M, Mustakallio KK. The fine structure of the spindle cell in Kaposi's sarcoma. Arch Pathol Microbiol Scand 1965; 63:567–75.
54. Harrison AC, Kahn LB. Myogenic cells in Kaposi's sarcoma: an ultrastructural study. J Pathol 1978; 124:157–60.
55. Waldo ED, Vuletin JC, Kay GI. The ultrastructure of vascular tumors. Additional observations and a review of the literature. Pathol Annu 1979; 12 (2):279.
56. Dorfman RF. The ultrastructure of Kaposi's sarcoma. Lab Invest 1964; 13:939.
57. McNutt NC, Fletcher V, Conant MA. Early lesions of Kaposi's sarcoma in homosexual men. An ultrastructural comparison with other vascular proliferations in skin. Am J Pathol 1983; 111:62–77.
58. Schmoekel C, Braun-Falco O. Der atypische morbus Kaposi. Hauterzt 1976; 27:291–5.
59. Fawcett DW. In: Orbison JL, Smith D, eds. Comparative Observations on the Fine Structure of Blood Capillaries. The Peripheral Blood Vessel. Baltimore, Williams & Wilkins, 1963:17–44
60. Leak LV. The structure of lymphatic capillaries in lymph formation. Fed Proc 1976; 35:1863–71.
61. Guarda LG, Silva EG, Ordonez NG, Smith JL Jr. Factor VIII in Kaposi's sarcoma. Am J Clin Pathol 1981; 76:197–200.

62. Nadji M, Morales AR, Ziegles-Weissman J, Penneys NS. Kaposi's sarcoma. Immunohistologic evidence for an endothelial origin. Arch Pathol Lab Med 1981; 105:274–5.
63. Walter PR, Philippe E, Nguemby-Mbina C, Chamlian A. Kaposi's sarcoma: presence of herpes-type virus particles in a tumor specimen. Hum Pathol 1984; 15:1145–6.
64. Kopf AW. The distribution of alkaline phosphatase in normal and pathologic human skin. AMA Arch Dermatol 1957; 75:1–37.
65. Sternberger LA. Immunocytochemistry. 2d ed. New York, Wiley, 1979.
66. Millard ER, Heryet AR. An immunohistological study of factor VIII-related antigen and Kaposi's sarcoma using polyclonal and monoclonal antibodies. J Pathol 1985; 146:31–8.
67. Sehested M, Hou-Jensen K. Factor VIII-related antigen as an endothelial cell marker in benign and malignant diseases. Virchows Arch (Pathol Anat) 1981; 391:217–25.
68. Svanholm H, Karsten N, Hauge P. Factor VIII-related antigen and lymphatic collecting vessels. Virchows Arch (Pathol Anat) 1984; 404:223–8.
69. Mason DY, Biberfeld P. Technical aspects of lymphoma immunohistochemistry. J Histochem Cytochem 1980; 28:731–45.
70. Wilson AJ. Factor VIII-related antigen staining by immunoperoxidase technique in smaller laboratories: a potential problem. Am Clin Pathol 1984; 81:117–20.
71. Olweny CLM, Kaddumukasa A, Atine L, Owor R, Magrath I, Ziegler JL. Childhood Kaposi's sarcoma: clinical features and therapy. Br J Cancer 1976; 33:555–60.
72. Burns BF, Wood GS, Dorfman RF. The varied histopathology of lymphadenopathy in the homosexual male. Am J Surg Pathol 1985; 9:287–97.
73. Gottlieb G, Ackerman AB. Kaposi's sarcoma. An extensively disseminated form in young homosexual men. Hum Pathol 1982; 13:882–92.
74. Rutgers JL, Wieczorek R, Bonetti F, Kaplan KL, Posnet DN, Friedman-Kien AE, Knowles DM. The expression of endothelial cell surface antigens by AIDS-associated Kaposi's sarcoma. Evidence for a vascular endothelial cell origin. Am J Pathol 1986; 122:493–9.
75. Turner RR, Beckstead JH, Warnke RA, Wood GS. Endothelial cell phenotypic diversity. In situ demonstration of immunologic and

enzymatic heterogeneity that correlates with specific morphologic subtypes. Am J Clin Pathol (in press).
76. Bendelac A, Kanitakis J, Chouvet B, Thivolet J. Basement membrane in Kaposi's sarcoma: an immunohistochemical and ultrastructural study. Pathol Res Pract 1985; 180:626–32.
77. Kramer RH, Fuh GM, Hwang CBC, Conant MA, Greenspan JS. Basement membrane and connective tissue proteins in early lesions of Kaposi's sarcoma associated with AIDS. J Invest Dermatol 1985; 84:516–20.
78. Barsky SH, Baker A, Siegal GP, Togo S, Liotta LA. Use of anti-basement membrane antibodies to distinguish blood vessel capillaries from lymphatic capillaries. Am J Surg Pathol 1983B; 7:667–77.
79. Jones RR, Spaul J, Spry C, Wilson Jones E. Histogenesis of Kaposi's sarcoma in patients with and without acquired immune deficiency syndrome (AIDS). J Clin Pathol 1986; 39:742–9.
80. Spence IM. Growth in vitro of a strain of cells derived from a Kaposi tumor. Acta Union Int Contre Cancer 1962; 18:490–3.
81. Davison PM, Bensch K, Karasek MA. Isolation and growth of endothelial cells from the microvessels of the newborn human foreskin in cell culture. J Invest Dermatol 1980; 75:316–21.
82. Bensch KG, Davison PM, Karasek MA. Factors controlling the in vitro growth pattern of human microvascular endothelial cells. J Ultrastruct Res 1983; 82:76–89.
83. Karasek MA. Personal communication. 1987.
84. Fenoglio CM, Oster M, LoGerfo P, et al. Kaposi's sarcoma following chemotherapy for testicular cancer in a homosexual man: demonstration of cytomegalovirus RNA in sarcoma cells. Hum Pathol 1982; 13:955–9.
85. Cerimele D, Scappaticci S, Cattaneo E, Cottoni F. Failure to demonstrate early and late antigens of cytomegalovirus in tissue cultures from Kaposi's sarcoma patients. Arch Dermatol Res 1983; 275:197–8.
86. Oettlé AG. Geographical and racial differences in the frequency of Kaposi's sarcoma as evidence of environmental and genetic causes. Acta Union Int Contre Cancer 1962; 18:330–63.
87. Oettlé AG, Kaminer B. Failure to grow Kaposi's sarcoma tissue in mouse brain. Acta Union Int Contre Cancer 1962; 18:487.
88. Becker SW, Thatcher HW. Multiple idiopathic hemorrhagic sarcoma of Kaposi; historical review, nomenclature and theories rele-

vant to the nature of the disease with experimental studies of two cases. J Invest Dermatol 1939; 1:379–89.

89. Lo SC, Liotta LA. Vascular tumors produced by NIH/3T3 cells transfected with human AIDS Kaposi's sarcoma DNA. Am J Pathol 1985; 118:7–13.
90. Costa J, Rabson AS. Generalized Kaposi's sarcoma is not a neoplasm. Lancet 1983; 1:58.
91. Cleary ML, Sklar J. Lymphoproliferative disorders in cardiac transplant recipients are multiclonal lymphomas. Lancet 1984; 1:489–93.
92. Cleary ML, Dorfman RF, Sklar J. Failure in immunological control of the virus infection: post-transplant lymphomas. In: Epstein MA, Achong BC, eds. The Epstein-Barr Virus: Recent Advances. London, William Heinemann Medical Books 1986: 164–81.

4

Etiology: Role of Cytomegalovirus

W. Lawrence Drew
Mount Zion Hospital and Medical Center
San Francisco, California

Eng-shang Huang
Lineberger Cancer Research Center
University of North Carolina
Chapel Hill, North Carolina

The first evidence of an association between Kaposi's sarcoma and cytomegalovirus (CMV) was presented by Giraldo and Beth and colleagues in 1972 (1,2). They isolated a unique strain, K9V, from a cell line derived from a Kaposi's sarcoma patient from Zaire. This strain shared significant homology with another transforming CMV strain, Mj, and was capable of inducing lymphadenopathy in young baboons. This discovery began a continuing search for evidence that CMV plays a causal role in the genesis of Kaposi's sarcoma. This chapter chronicles that search.

MOLECULAR VIROLOGY

The potential for CMV to be an oncogenic virus has been the subject of several reviews (3,4). As summarized in Table 1, the virus stimulates the synthesis of cellular DNA, RNA, and enzymes in host cells (5,6). CMV transforms human embryo fibroblasts, which then grow as sarcomatous tumors when transplanted to immunosuppressed or athymic mice (7). Nelson et al. (8) have refined the latter observation by identifying the transforming segment of the CMV genome. Additionally, Stinski and Roehr (9) and Boshart et al. (10) have shown that the gene products responsible for immediate-early antigen coding can activate transcription. We have demonstrated that the immediate-early gene region of human CMV stimulated the transcription of human immunodeficiency virus (HIV) (Davis MG, et al. submitted for publication). This stimulation could enhance HIV replication, for example, in patients with the acquired immunodeficiency syndrome (AIDS) with a previous or concurrent human CMV infection.

The second line of evidence linking CMV to Kaposi's sarcoma stems from work reported previously by Giraldo et al. (11). A significantly higher prevalence of CMV antibody was detected in 46 elderly European and U.S. patients with Kaposi's sarcoma than in two age-matched control groups without Kaposi's sarcoma. This serologic difference was not seen with antibodies to the Epstein-Barr virus (EBV), herpes simplex virus (HSV), and varicella zoster virus. No differences in serologic patterns were observed in African

Table 1 Oncogenic Potential of Human Cytomegalovirus In Vitro

Stimulation of cellular macromolecule synthesis
Cellular DNA
Cellular RNA
Mitochondrial DNA
Cellular enzymes
DNA polymerase (α and β)
Thymidine kinase
Ornithine decarboxylase
Plasminogen activator
DNA-dependent RNA polymerase
Exonuclease
Topoisomerase
Morphological transformation of mammalian cells
Hamster embryonic fibroblast
Rodent cells
Human fibroblast

Source: After Reference 18, Table 2.

Kaposi's sarcoma patients versus controls because of a high background of CMV seropositivity (12).

Further evidence for an association of CMV with Kaposi's sarcoma derives from the demonstration of CMV nucleic acids and antigens in Kaposi's sarcoma tumor biopsies. Reports of detection of CMV antigens, DNA, or RNA in Kaposi's sarcoma tissue are conflicting. Boldogh et al. (13) and Giraldo et al. (14) have reported the presence of CMV early antigens in tumor tissues from patients with classic and endemic forms of Kaposi's sarcoma. We have detected CMV early antigens by a similar procedure in 6 of 9 Kaposi's sarcoma biopsy specimens from homosexual men with AIDS (15) and more recently have found this antigen in an additional 9 of 18 cases examined. Biopsies of normal skin from 21 of 22 of our patients were negative for CMV antigens, and all Kaposi's sarcoma biopsies were also negative for CMV by culture. The

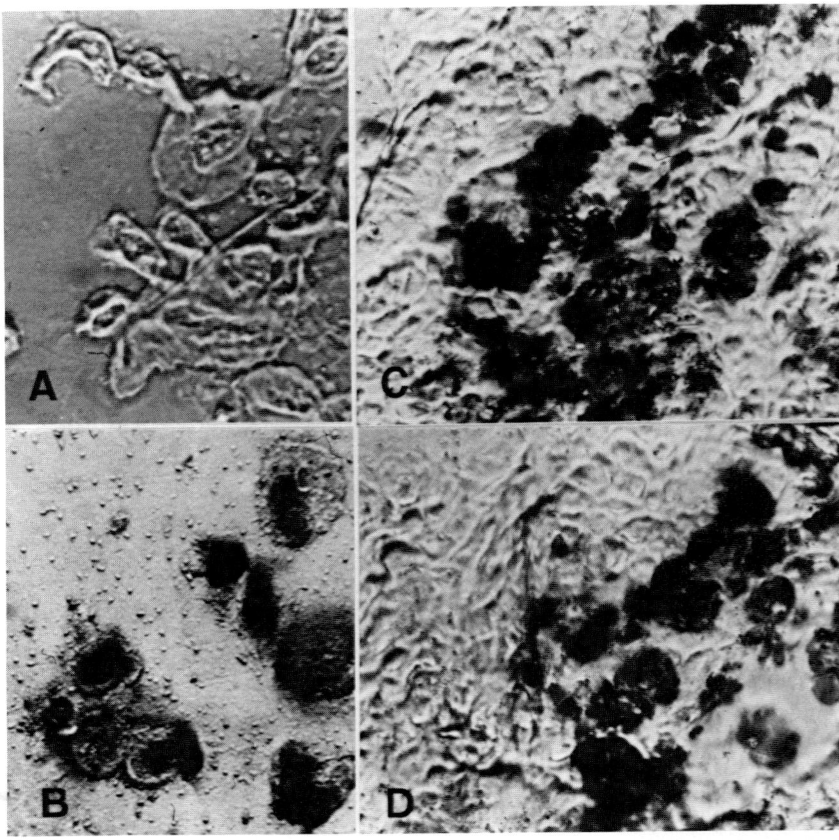

Figure 1 Demonstration of CMV DNA and RNA in tumor cells in lymph node from Kaposi's sarcoma patient (22) by in situ nucleic acid hybridization using biotinylated CMV DNA as probe (C and D). Mock-infected (A) and virus-infected (B) WI-38 human fibroblasts were used for comparison. Virus-infected cells were harvested 72 hours after infection by trypsinization. (Reproduced from Reference 12, Figure 4.)

presence of CMV early antigens, coupled with the failure to detect CMV late antigens or whole virus in Kaposi's sarcoma biopsies (14,16), suggests that CMV genome is present in a nonreplicative (and hence more likely oncogenic) state and rules out the possibility that viral presence results simply from disseminated CMV infection or from a tropism of the virus for dermal or tumor tissue.

Boldogh et al. (13) have also detected CMV DNA in 6 of 12, and CMV RNA in 3 of 9 biopsies from African patients. EBV and HSV type 2 sequences were not detected. We reported the presence of CMV RNA by in situ hybridization in 2 of 3 Kaposi's sarcoma biopsies from homosexual men whose tumor cultures were negative for replicating CMV (17). We have also demonstrated viral nucleic acid and in tumor cell foci in lymph nodes of Kaposi's sarcoma patients by in situ nucleic acid hybridization using biotinylated DNA as probe (Figure 1) (5).

More recently, Spector et al. (18) have employed the technique of in situ hybridization to detect CMV DNA specifically within tumor cells of Kaposi's sarcoma tissue specimens. Instead of whole virus genome, they used as probes subgenomic fragments of CMV DNA that had been shown previously not to cross-hybridize with host cell human DNA. With this technique they were able to detect CMV genetic sequences in tumor cells from 6 of 10 evaluable Kaposi's sarcoma specimens but not in sections of uninvolved skin (18). Others have been unable to detect CMV DNA or RNA in Kaposi's sarcoma tumor tissue (16,19). In part this may stem from the use of procedures of differing sensitivity. For example, using a Southern blot procedure, Ruger et al. were not able to detect CMV DNA in 6 AIDS-related Kaposi's sarcoma tissues they examined. In biopsies from 8 African patients and 1 European Kaposi's sarcoma patient, they detected marginal hybridization in only 2 (19).

EPIDEMIOLOGY

The epidemiologic evidence for CMV involvement in Kaposi's sarcoma derives from the heightened prevalence of this tumor in two groups of individuals, renal transplant patients and homosexual men with AIDS, who share the dual features of immunosuppression and extremely high rates of active CMV infection.

CMV in Renal Transplant Patients

There have been at least 36 reports of Kaposi's sarcoma in renal transplant patients (20,21); it is estimated that Kaposi's sarcoma accounts for more than 3% of all malignancies in organ transplant recipients (see Chapter 5) (22). Although specific CMV studies have not been reported in these patients, renal transplant recipients as a group are subject to extremely high rates of primary or reactivated CMV infection (23), and all these patients are, of course, immunosuppressed during the posttransplant period. Kaposi's sarcoma appears an average of 16–36 months after transplantation, suggesting an approximate incubation period for the development of the tumor in immunocompromised patients.

CMV in Homosexual Men

The initial documentation of high rates of CMV infection in homosexual men resulted from prevalence studies we performed at the San Francisco City Clinic in 1979 (24). We observed urinary excretion of CMV in 14 of 90 (7.4%). homosexual men, but in none of 101 heterosexual men attending the same sexually transmitted disease clinic ($p < 0.005$). Similarly, antibody to CMV was detected in 130 of 139 (93.5%) homosexuals but in only 38 of 70 (54.3%) heterosexual men ($p < 0.005$).

In a subsequent prospective study of homosexual men participating in the Western Study Group Hepatitis Vaccine Trial at the San Francisco City Clinic, we again noted a high prevalence of CMV IgG serum antibody in 206 of 237 men, or 86.9% (25). Of the 31 men lacking CMV antibody on initial testing, 22 experienced seroconversion within 9 months of follow-up, for an attack rate of 71% during this time period.

During a mean follow-up period of 14.3 months (range 2–20);

66 of the 206 initially seropositive men (32%) excreted CMV in their urine on one or more occasions. Both a urine and a semen specimen were obtained during a single visit from 52 of the homosexual men. CMV was recovered from 18 of the semen specimens but from only 3 of the 18 corresponding urine samples. Specimens from a single individual grew CMV from the urine but not from the semen. Semen would therefore appear to be nearly five times as sensitive as urine in detecting the presence of CMV. In our study of CMV infection among asymptomatic homosexual males in the Research Triangle area in North Carolina, we found that CMV could be isolated repeatedly from semen specimens of 13 of 40 (30%) of homosexual males examined. Virus could be demonstrated inside the sperm head as well as in the extracellular seminal fluid (5,26). Clearly, the widespread occurrence of CMV in urine and semen in this population makes exposure to the virus all but inevitable and accounts for the extraordinarily high attack rate of CMV infections among seronegative homosexual men.

Data on the prevalence of CMV IgM antibody further suggest that homosexuals experience repeated episodes of CMV infections. CMV IgM antibody was detected on one or more occasions in the sera of more than 90% of the homosexual men and tended to appear, disappear, and then reappear again over the course of time (25). In contrast, IgM antibody to CMV was detected in only 2.8% of 103 serum specimens randomly collected from volunteer male blood donors. Among the homosexual men there was no temporal correlation between the presence of CMV viruria and serum IgM antibody titers. CMV IgM antibody was detected in a significantly ($p < 0.05$) higher proportion of serum samples from the 206 initially seropositive men (67% of 1135 samples) than in the postconversion samples obtained from the 22 seroconverters (53% of 86 samples). These data are summarized in Table 2. The higher prevalence of CMV IgM antibody in long-standing seropositive men than in recent seroconverters suggests that the former group is continually re-exposed to (and possibly reinfected with) exogenous strains of the virus. We have determined recently that this CMV-specific IgM antibody reflects reinfection in at least some

Table 2 Presence of CMV IgM Antibody in 237 Prospectively Studied Homosexual Men

Group	Subjects, no. positive/ no. tested (%)	Serum samples,[a] no. positive/ no. tested (%)
Seronegatives	0/9 (0)	0/54 (0)
Seropositives	196/206 (95)	165/1136 (67)
Seroconverters	20/22 (91)	46/86 (53)[b]

[a]Serial sera collected over a 3-year period of follow-up.
[b]Samples obtained after seroconversion.

patients. Using a restriction enzyme technique to distinguish different isolates, we found that four of four AIDS patients had at least two different CMV isolates from their autopsy organ cultures.

To date, we have studied 57 homosexual men with Kaposi's sarcoma for CMV antibody, and all are positive. Of 39 who have had appropriate secretion cultures, 24 (62%) have been positive. Zur Hausen (27) has stated, "it is likely that the epigenetic burden of persisting viral DNA increases with the number of infections and is therefore correlated with age and exposure." Consistent with this hypothesis are our observations that the average age of homosexual men with Kaposi's sarcoma is 36 years and that they have been homosexual for an average of 17 years (28). A quantitative estimate of the extent of CMV exposure among homosexual men can be inferred from the finding that, even on a single sample, the semen of 25% of homosexual men is CMV culture positive (25).

CMV in Intravenous Drug Users

A most important epidemiologic clue linking CMV to Kaposi's sarcoma has come to light during the current AIDS epidemic: the marked discrepancy in the incidence of Kaposi's sarcoma cases among homosexual versus heterosexual AIDS patients. In New York City, Kaposi's sarcoma occurs in 46% of AIDS cases among homosexual men but in only 3.8% of AIDS cases among heterosexual men (28). This striking difference suggests that a cofactor may be present in homosexual men that is not present in heterosexuals. This cofactor may be CMV infection since intravenous (IV) drug users (most of whom are heterosexual) do not have unusually high rates of CMV infection. Of 143 IV drug users in San Francisco and New York City, only 92 (64%) were seropositive, a rate similar to that observed in the general population (29). Marmor et al. have extended this observation to compare the prevalence of CMV antibody in IV drug-using women (87%) versus men (42%) (30). This finding adds to the correlation of CMV antibody and Kaposi's sarcoma prevalence since Kaposi's sarcoma is more common as the presenting manifestation of AIDS in IV drug-using women (Kaposi's sarcoma prevalence 12.5%) than in IV drug-using men (3.8%) (28). Table 3, based on their report, shows that the prevalence of Kaposi's sarcoma as a presenting manifestation of AIDS

Table 3 Relationship Between CMV Seropositivity and Kaposi's Sarcoma in AIDS Patients

AIDS risk group	CMV seropositive (%)	Kaposi's Sarcoma in initial diagnosis (%)[a]
Homosexual/bisexual	94[b]	46[a]
Females with IV drug use	87[c]	12.5[a]
Males with IV drug use	42[c]–64[d]	3.8[a]

[a]DeJarlais et al. N Engl J Med 1984; 310:1119.
[b]Drew et al. J Infect Dis 1981; 143:188–92.
[c]Marmor et al. Int. Conf. on AIDS, April 1985.
[d]Brodie et al. AIDS Memorandum, vol. 1(7), 1984.

correlates generally with the prevalence of CMV antibody in the risk group. The use of CMV IgG antibody prevalence is an imperfect marker of the magnitude of CMV exposures in a group such as homosexual men. In this group, as documented previously, there may be multiple, repetitive exposures and even infection by the virus yet antibody measures only a single exposure (31).

CHANGES IN INCIDENCE OF AIDS-ASSOCIATED KAPOSI'S SARCOMA

Most recently a decline has been noted in Kaposi's sarcoma as the presenting manifestation of AIDS in homosexual men. As shown in Figure 2, we have been able to relate this decline to a similar decline in the acquisition of CMV infection among seronegative homosexual men. As mentioned previously, 22 of 31 (71%) homosexual men who were CMV seronegative acquired infection during the first 7 months of 1981. In contrast, only 1 of 26 CMV seronegative men acquired CMV during the 12 months of 1984. Correspondingly, the prevalence of Kaposi's sarcoma as the presenting manifestation of AIDS in homosexual men has declined from 63% in 1981 to 24% in 1985.

The reason for the decline in CMV infections is undoubtedly the reduction of sexually transmitted disease, in general, among homosexual men. At least in San Francisco, the rates of gonorrhea, amebiasis, and other such diseases have diminished during the past 2 years in association with the closure of bathhouses and adoption of "safe sex" guidelines.

The decline in Kaposi's sarcoma may reflect diminished exposure to any one or several sexually transmitted diseases, as well as to other putative cofactors, such as amyl nitrite, which is used to assist the frequency of sexual acts (32). Thus, the correlation of decreased Kaposi's sarcoma with decreased CMV infection may be only coincidental. However, in view of the many threads of evidence implicating CMV in Kaposi's sarcoma, the observation is provocative.

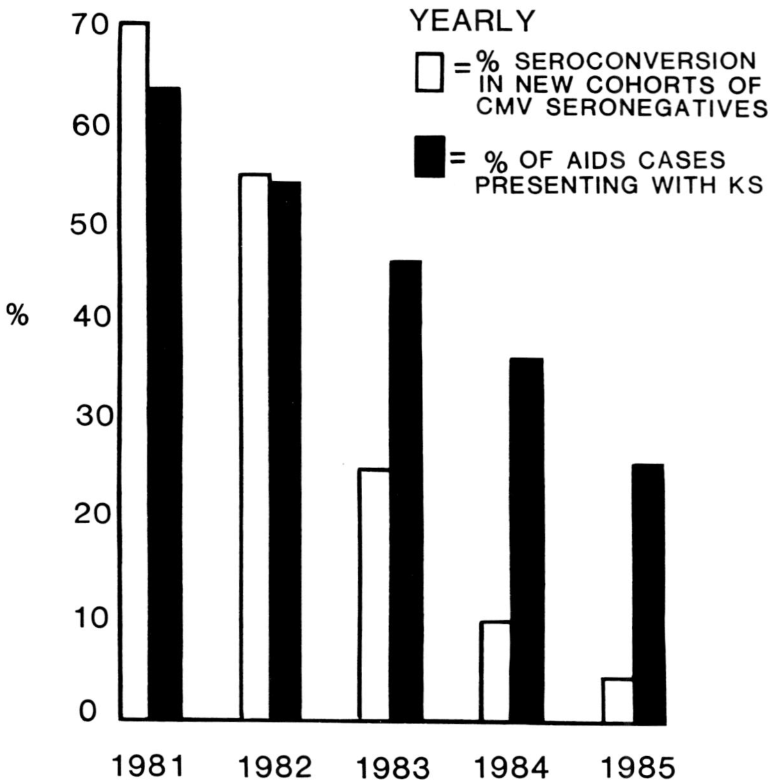

Figure 2 Incidence of Kaposi's sarcoma in AIDS in San Francisco from 1981 through 1985 (G. Rutherford, personal communication) compared with rate of CMV seroconversion observed in seronegative homosexual men over the same time period (L. Drew, unpublished data).

SUMMARY

An etiologic role for CMV in the pathogenesis of Kaposi's sarcoma has yet to be established. As mentioned in this review and by others (Chapters 1, 5 and 6) (3,4), several possibilities exist. These are outlined in Figure 3. The transforming sequences in CMV may immortalize its endothelial target cell in a manner analogous to the

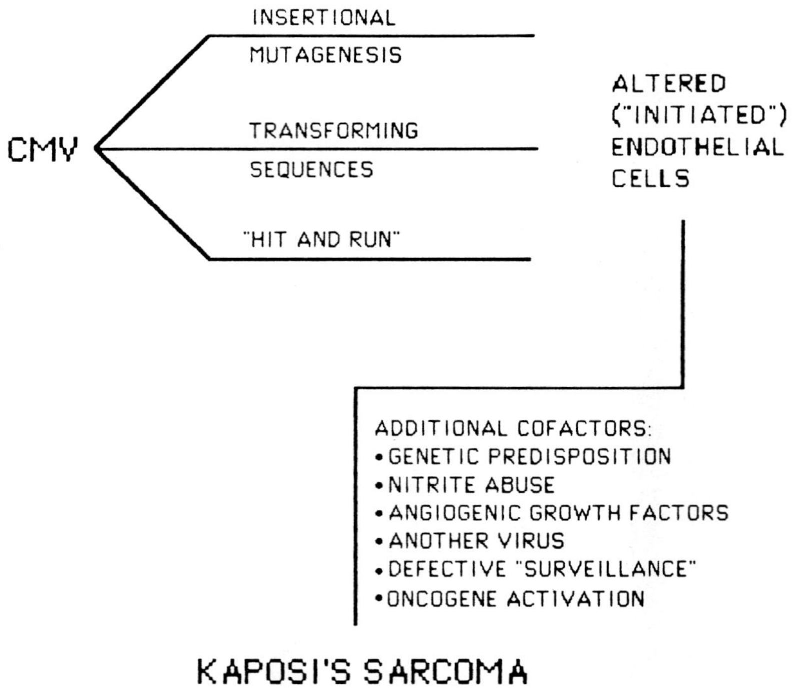

Figure 3 Speculative roles of cytomegalovirus in the pathogenesis of Kaposi's sarcoma include various mechanisms of viral alteration of cellular gene regulation or funtion. Insertional mutagenesis occurs when viral genes increase the risk of host DNA mutations; viral transforming sequences or promotor regions may alter the proliferative potential of the host cell; finally, a "hit-and-run" mechanism may explain how cells can become "initiated" by virus when no trace of the virus can later be found. Obviously, other cofactors that impinge on cell proliferation and autonomy must interact between the viral alteration of the endothelial cell and evolution to a malignant phenotype.

transforming effects of Epstein-Barr virus on B lymphocytes (33). Alternatively, CMV may induce a state of "insertional mutagenesis" by integrating powerful regulatory genes into the target cell (34). Or, CMV may interact with an additional cofactor (such as angiogenesis factor) to induce its proliferative effects. The failure to detect CMV genome or antigen in all cases of Kaposi's sarcoma has two possible explanations: the virus produces its effects by a "hit-and-run" mechanism, or the virus has no etiologic relationship in some cases of Kaposi's sarcoma. As indicated in Figure 3, other cofactors must be postulated to interact with CMV-infected endothelial cells to induce the malignant phenotype. Clearly, the association of CMV as a putative cofactor in Kaposi's sarcoma cannot be ignored; future research may be aided by the development of an animal model (35) and through the use of endothelial tissue cultures derived from malignant tumors (36).

REFERENCES

1. Giraldo G, Beth E, Coeur P, Vogel CL, Dhru DS. Kaposi's sarcoma: a new model in the search for viruses associated with human malignancies. JNCI 1972; 49:1495–1507.
2. Giraldo G, Beth E, Hagenau F. Herpes-type virus particles in tissue culture of Kaposi's sarcoma from different geographic regions. JNCI 1972; 49:1509–13.
3. Giraldo G, Beth E, Buonaguro FM. Kaposi's sarcoma: a natural model of interrelationships between viruses, immunologic responses, genetics, and oncogenesis. Antibiot Chemother 1984; 32:1–11.
4. Spector DH, Spector SA. The oncogenic potential of human cytomegalovirus. Prog Med Virol 1984; 29:45–89.
5. Huang ES. The role of cytomegalovirus infection in Kaposi's sarcoma. In Friedman-Kien AE, Laubenstein LJ, eds. AIDS—The Epidemic of Kaposi's Sarcoma and Opportunistic Infections. Masson Publishing, 1984:111–26.
6. St Jeor SC, Albrecht TB, Frank FD, Rapp R. Stimulation of cellular DNA synthesis with human cytomegalovirus. J Virol 1974; 13:353–62.

7. Geder L, Lausch R, O'Neill F, Rapp F. Oncogenic transformation of human embryo lung cells by human cytomegalovirus. Science 1976; 192:1134–7.
8. Nelson J, Fleckenstein B, Galloway DA, McDougall JK. Transformation of NIH3T3 cells with cloned fragments of human cytomegalovirus AD-169. J Virol 1982; 43:83.
9. Stinski MF, Roehr T. Activation of the major immediate early gene of human cytomegalovirus by cis-acting elements in the promoter regulatory sequence and by virus-specific trans-acting components. J Virol 1985; 55:431–41.
10. Boshart M, Weber F, Gerhard J, Dorsch-Hasler K, Fleckenstein B, Schaffer W. A strong enhancer is located upstream of an immediate early gene of human cytomegalovirus. Cell 1985; 41:521–30.
11. Giraldo G, Beth E, Henle W, et al. Antibody patterns to herpesviruses in Kaposi's sarcoma. II. Serological association of American Kaposi's sarcoma with cytomegalovirus. Int J Cancer 1978; 22:126–31.
12. Giraldo G, Beth E, Kourilsky FM, Henle W, Henle G, Miké V, Huraus JM, Andersen HK, Gharbi MR, Kyalwazi SK, Puissant A. Antibody patterns of herpesviruses in Kaposi's sarcoma: serologic association of European Kaposi's sarcoma with cytomegalovirus. Int J Cancer 1975; 15:839–48.
13. Boldogh I, Beth E, Huang E-S, Kyalwazi SK, Giraldo G. Kaposi's sarcoma. IV. Detection of CMV DNA, CMV RNA, and CMNA in tumour biopsies. Int J Cancer 1981; 28:469–74.
14. Giraldo G, Beth E, Huang E-S. Kaposi's sarcoma and its relationship to cytomegalovirus (CMV). III. CMV DNA and CMV-early antigens in Kaposi's sarcoma. Int J Cancer 1980; 26:23–9.
15. Drew WL, Conant MA, Miner RC, et al. Cytomegalovirus and Kaposi's sarcoma in young homosexual men. Lancet 1982; 2:125–7.
16. Civantos F, Penneys NS, Haines H. Kaposi's sarcoma: absence of cytomegalovirus. J Invest Dermatol 1982; 79:79–80.
17. Stribling J, Weitzner S, Smith GV. Kaposi's sarcoma in renal allograft recipients. Cancer 1978; 42:442–6.
18. Spector DH, Shaw SB, Hock LJ, et al. Association of human cytomegalovirus with Kaposi's sarcoma. In Gottlieb MS, Groopman JE, eds. Acquired Immune Deficiency Syndrome. New York, Alan R. Liss, 1984:109–26.
19. Ruger R, Burmester GR, Kalden JR, Bienzle U, Braun R, Safai B,

Sterry W, Fleckenstein B. Search for human cytomegalovirus DNA in Kaposi's sarcomas and hematopoietic cells from homosexual men with AIDS or unexplained lymphadenopathy. In Gottlieb MS, Groopman JE, eds. Acquired Immune Deficiency Syndrome. New York, Alan R. Liss, 1984:127–37.

20. Myers BD, Kessler E, Levi J, Pick A, Rosenfeld JB, Tikvah P. Kaposi's sarcoma in kidney transplant recipients. Arch Intern Med 1974; 133:307–11.
21. Harwood AR, Osoba D, Hofstader SL, et al. Kaposi's sarcoma in recipients of renal transplants. Am J Med 1979; 67:759–65.
22. Penn I. Kaposi's sarcoma in organ transplant recipients. Transplantation 1979; 27:8–11.
23. Fiala M, Payne JE, Berne TV, et al. Epidemiology of cytomegalovirus infection after transplantation and immunosuppression. J Infect Dis 1975; 132:421–32.
24. Drew WL, Mintz L, Miner RC, Sands M, Ketterer B. Prevalence of cytomegalovirus infection in homosexual men. J Infect Dis 1981; 143:188–92.
25. Mintz L, Drew WL, Miner RC, Braff EH. Cytomegalovirus infections in homosexual men: an epidemiological study. Ann Intern Med 1983; 99:326–9.
26. Huang ES, Davis MG, Baskear JF, Huong SM. Molecular epidemiology and oncogenicity of human cytomegalovirus. In: Harris CC, ed. Biochemical and Molecular Biology of Cancer. UCLA Symposium on Molecular and Cellular Biology. New Series 1986; 40:323–44.
27. Zur Hausen H. The role of viruses in human tumors. Adv Cancer Res 1980; 33:77–107.
28. De Jarlais DC, Marmor M, Thomas P, Chamberland M, Zolla-Pazner S, Sencer DJ. N Engl J Med 1984; 310:1119.
29. Brodie HR, Drew WL, Maayan S. Prevalence of Kaposi's sarcoma in AIDS patients reflects differences in rates of cytomegalovirus infection in high risk groups. AIDS Memorandum 1984; 1(7):12.
30. Marmor M, Des Jarlais DC, Spira T, et al. AIDS and cytomegalovirus exposure in New York City drug abusers. International Conference on AIDS, Atlanta, Georgia, April 1985:52 (poster).
31. Drew WL, Mocarski ES, Sweet E, Miner RC. Multiple infections with CMV in AIDS patients: documentation by southern blot hybridization. J Infect Dis 1984; 150:952.
32. McKusick L, Horstman W, Coates TJ. AIDS and sexual behavior

reported by gay men in San Francisco. Am J Public Health 1985; 75:493–6.
33. Kieff E, Dambaugh T, Hummel M, Keller M. Epstein-Barr virus transformation and replication. Adv Virol 1983; 3:133–82.
34. Bishop M. The molecular genetics of cancer. Nature 1986; 235:305–11.
35. Sato N, Sato T, Takahashi S, Kikuchi K. Establishment of murine endothelial cell lines that develop angiosarcomas in vivo: brief demonstration of a proposed animal model for Kaposi's sarcoma. Cancer Res 1986; 46:362–6.
36. Robinson RA, Ten Eyck CJ, Hart MN. Establishment and preliminary growth characteristics of a transformed mouse cerebral microvessel endothelial cell line. Lab Invest 1986; 54:579–88.

5

Etiology: Immunodeficiency

Israel Penn
University of Cincinnati Medical Center
and Veterans Administration Medical Center
Cincinnati, Ohio

Until recently Kaposi's sarcoma was a rare malignancy in Europe and the United States. The annual incidence was estimated as 0.021–0.061 per 100,000 people (1,2). Kaposi's sarcoma comprised 0.02–0.07% of all cancers in the United States (3,4). Among whites it occurred mostly in Jews of Central and Eastern European origin and among persons of Southern European ancestry (4). The disease was frequently referred to as classic or European Kaposi's sarcoma. Among blacks the incidence was at least as common and may possibly have been higher than in white Americans. However, the incidence in American blacks was many times less than in African blacks (3). The disease seen in the general population of the United States occurred predominantly among elderly men, ran an indolent course of 8–13 years, and seldom caused death (5). Typically the lesions appeared on the lower extremities, and clinical evidence of lymph node and visceral involvement was uncommon. However, at autopsy internal involvement, particularly gastrointestinal, was present quite frequently. Spontaneous regression of lesions occurred in approximately 2% of patients (3).

In recent years there has been a substantial increase in the incidence of Kaposi's sarcoma in certain population groups (6–14). Considerable evidence has accumulated indicating that immunologic deficiencies may play an important role in the pathogenesis and progression of Kaposi's sarcoma in these people. In this chapter, we consider four categories of patients: individuals with the acquired immunodeficiency syndrome (AIDS) who have epidemic Kaposi's sarcoma; African patients who have endemic Kaposi's sarcoma; organ transplant recipients with Kaposi's sarcoma; and immunosuppressed nonorgan transplant patients with Kaposi's sarcoma. In addition, the role of immunodeficiency in causing Kaposi's sarcoma will be discussed.

ACQUIRED IMMUNODEFICIENCY SYNDROME

This syndrome consists of complex, profound, and perhaps irreversible abnormalities in cellular immune function associated with opportunistic infections and aggressive neoplasms, mostly Kaposi's sarcoma and non-Hodgkin's lymphomas (NHL) (10,11,14). The major immunologic defect affects T helper-inducer cells, but B-cell abnormalities are also present (11). The most characteristic findings include lymphopenia, reduced T helper-T suppressor cell ratios due to a reduction in the absolute numbers of T-helper cells, and cutaneous anergy. Patients with AIDS are afflicted by a wide variety of opportunistic pathogens, including protozoa, yeasts, bacteria, and viruses. Evidence of infection by cytomegalovirus (CMV), Epstein-Barr virus (EBV), and hepatitis B virus is frequently found.

AIDS occurs in socially, ethnically, and genetically diverse hosts (11,14). The major affected group consists of homosexual men, particularly those with numerous, anonymous sexual contacts. Others include intravenous drug abusers, hemophiliac patients, recipients of random blood transfusions, female sexual partners of persons with the syndrome, Haitian immigrants to the United States, Central Africans, and children of mothers at high risk for the syndrome (11,14,15). A small percentage of patients do not fall into any known risk category.

AIDS is caused by the HTLV-III (human T-lymphotropic virus type III), also known as LAV (lymphadenopathy virus). The causative retrovirus is now named human immunodeficiency virus (HIV). It is believed that various cofactors impair immunity and play a role in permitting the infection to become established and to devastate the immune system (11,14,16). These include multiple viral infections; exposure to foreign antigens, such as blood products, or allogeneic sperm and semen, particularly in the anoreceptive sexual partner; abuse of intravenous drugs; the use of volatile nitrites; and exposure to HLA alloantigens that can induce immune suppression as a result of donor recognition of host major compatibility complex (MHC) antigens (graft versus host) and/or host recognition of donor MHC antigens (host versus graft); and lack of natural resistance as may occur in infants (11,14,16).

The risk of development of Kaposi's sarcoma in AIDS patients is approximately 100 times greater than that in the general population (17). By June 9, 1986, a total of 21,517 cases of AIDS were reported to the Centers for Disease Control in Atlanta, Georgia. Kaposi's sarcoma was reported in 4093 male homosexuals or bisexuals and in 223 members of other risk groups. It is not clear why homosexual or bisexual men have a higher incidence of Kaposi's sarcoma in comparison with other AIDS risk groups. Another puzzling feature is that the national proportion of AIDS patients with Kaposi's sarcoma has dropped from 34% in 1981, when AIDS was first identified, to 14% at present. Perhaps this is due to the decline in some cofactor, possibly a result of safer sexual practices among male homosexuals and bisexuals.

Apparently there is a higher incidence of Kaposi's sarcoma in AIDS patients of Italian ancestry (18). This may be connected with the relative frequency of HLA-DR5 antigen in Italians, which may make them more prone to Kaposi's sarcoma (see below).

Kaposi's sarcoma in AIDS differs from the disease seen in elderly Americans and from the endemic Kaposi's sarcoma seen in adult men in equatorial Africa but has similarities to the Kaposi's sarcoma seen in African children (see below) (19). It involves the skin in the majority of patients. However, the cutaneous lesions frequently look different from those seen in classic Kaposi's sarcoma and are often overlooked or misdiagnosed (20). The early skin lesions may be mistaken for bruises, ecchymoses, insect bites, nevi, dermatofibromas, secondary syphilis, or lichen planus. In a few patients skin involvement is absent at the initial examination but appears later in the course of the disease. The skin lesions tend to be widely dispersed and may occur in unusual locations, such as the tip of the nose, the penis, and areas of previous trauma (9). The disease is occasionally symmetrical.

More than half the patients with skin involvement have one or more lesions in the gastrointestinal tract (14,20). The stomach, duodenum, and colon may be affected simultaneously, or the tumors may be localized at only one site. Gastrointestinal Kaposi's sarcoma may antedate the development of overt skin lesions. Considerable differences may be present in the degree of gastrointestinal and skin involvement (14). Some patients have only one or two skin lesions but many tumors in the gastrointestinal tract. Visceral involvement may be silent clinically, or occult chronic blood loss may occur. Kaposi's sarcoma may also cause overt gastrointestinal bleeding or intestinal obstruction (21). Some lesions may be missed on routine gastrointestinal contrast studies as they may be small, telangiectatic, flat, or slightly papular red or blue areas in the esophagus, stomach, duodenum, or colon. Such tumors are best diagnosed by upper or lower gastrointestinal endoscopy (20,22). Some lesions may be raised, sessile red nodules varying from several millimeters to a centimeter or more in diameter (14). Large tumors may have a central umbilication or ulceration. Histologic confirmation is difficult as the lesions are submucosal and cannot be reached readily with endoscopic pinch biopsy forceps (14).

Kaposi's sarcoma in AIDS frequently involves lymph nodes (20). Usually they are clinically obvious, but in one study 50% of 18 patients had previously unsuspected enlargement of mesenteric and retroperitoneal nodes demonstrated on abdominal computed tomographic (CT) scan (22). Other less commonly affected sites are the mucous membranes of the mouth, pharynx, anus, conjunctiva, liver, spleen, lungs, brain, testis, pancreas, aorta, and heart (9,14,20,21). In some instances Kaposi's sarcoma and NHL occur in the same patient and may even occur side by side in the same lymph node. Kaposi's sarcoma in AIDS may occur in virtually any organ (14).

The two factors that greatly affect the prognosis are the extent of the Kaposi's sarcoma and the presence of opportunistic infections. These factors are undoubtedly influenced by the severity of the underlying immunodeficiency. In one study, patients with limited cutaneous disease had 100% survival at 24 months, compared with those with generalized disease but without systemic signs of fever or weight loss (B symptoms) who had a 60% survival (12). Only 16% of patients with either B symptoms or opportunistic infections were alive at 24 months.

Spontaneous regression of cutaneous Kaposi's sarcoma occurred in 6 of 159 AIDS patients (3.8%) (23). Regressions occurred in patients with minimal tumor burdens, none of whom had a history of opportunistic infection before the development of Kaposi's sarcoma. In another report of a single case, cutaneous Kaposi's sarcoma regressed although the patient's AIDS deteriorated (24). The authors believe that their case represents either a true abortive Kaposi's sarcoma or a Kaposi-form evolution of nonspecific lesions.

ENDEMIC KAPOSI'S SARCOMA IN AFRICA

The disease is most common among the black population in the rain forest area of Central Africa, where it makes up 3–9% of all malignancies (3,25). In some areas it is 150–200 times more common than in North America (3). The incidence of Kaposi's sarcoma is not increased in Asians and whites living in Africa (3). The major focus is in the northeast part of the Congo Basin, and the frequency lessens with distance from this focus, although the decline is not uniform. African Kaposi's sarcoma predominates in males but occurs in a younger age group (25–40 years) than European Kaposi's sarcoma. The first symptom is usually edema of the feet and legs, followed by vascular nodules or plaques in the same areas. Spontaneous regression of nodules is common, but in many patients, after an interval of months or years, nodules grow rapidly and ulcerate to form florid tumors, or woody infiltration of one or more limbs may occur (26). Regression is usually achieved with chemotherapeutic agents, and patients live for several years before death from disseminated disease. This variety of Kaposi's sarcoma in Africa is not related to HIV infection (27).

Children between the ages of 1 and 10 years may present with widespread lymphadenopathy and involvement of the ocular tissues and salivary glands, with few or no skin lesions (13). Clinically the disease is indistinguishable from lymphoma (9), and a lymph node biopsy is necessary to make the diagnosis. This disseminated form of Kaposi's sarcoma pursues a fulminant and usually fatal course. Attempts to prolong life with chemotherapy have met with limited success.

Recently there has been a marked increase in an aggressive form of Kaposi's sarcoma clinically similar to that seen in AIDS patients in the United States. This occurred in Zambia and Uganda, both areas with a high prevalence of endemic Kaposi's sarcoma (26). The aggressive variety is similar to the endemic type histologically but occurs as plaques, involves the lymph nodes, internal organs, trunk, and face, and has a rapidly fatal course. Patients with the aggressive epidemic form of Kaposi's sarcoma in Africa are HIV antibody positive (19). This type of Kaposi's sarcoma is also probably related to immunosuppression, since a mixed group of endemic and aggressive Kaposi's sarcoma patients from Zambia had a lower average T helper-T suppressor lymphocyte ratio than controls (28), but the helper-suppressor ratio in the endemic form of African Kaposi's sarcoma is within normal limits.

In African patients lymphomas (see Discussion) are less frequently associated with Kaposi's sarcoma than in the classic type, perhaps because the average age of the patients is lower, the disease frequently has followed a malignant course, and follow-up is less satisfactory (3).

ORGAN TRANSPLANT RECIPIENTS

The incidence of Kaposi's sarcoma in renal transplant recipients is increased 400- to 500-fold over that seen in a control population of the same ethnic origin (4). By August 1986, the Cincinnati Transplant Tumor Registry (CTTR) collected data on 2635 organ transplant recipients with 2817 types of cancer that had arisen de novo after transplantation. Of these neoplasms, 103 (3.7%) were Kaposi's sarcoma (4,6–8,29). If we exclude nonmelanoma skin cancers and in situ carcinomas of the uterine cervix, which are omitted from most cancer statistics, then Kaposi's sarcoma made up 5.2% of all malignancies. This remarkably high incidence of Kaposi's sarcoma occurred in a collection of patients reported from 20 countries. The geographic areas represented were North America (42 patients), Mediterranean countries in Europe, Asia, and Africa (34 patients), Western and Northern Europe (excluding Mediterranean countries) (11 patients), South America (9 patients), South Africa (4 patients), and Australia (3 patients). Incomplete data are available concerning the racial and ethnic backgrounds of the patients. The major groups were Arab (15), black (14, 9 from the United States, 5 from Africa), Western and Northern European whites (13), Jewish (11, mostly from Israel), Italian (11), Greek (10), Turkish (3), Brazilian (3), Spanish (2), Portuguese (2), and Mexican (2).

Two patients were heart transplant recipients and the remainder received renal allografts. The average age of the patients at the time of transplantation was 40.4 years (range 18–62 years), a very similar average age to that of the entire series of 2635 patients (average age 39.8 years). There were 71 males and 32 females. The 2:1 male-female ratio is much less than that seen in patients with classic Kaposi's sarcoma in whom it ranges from 9:1 to 15:1 (3,6,8).

All donors were free of cancer. Transplants were received from related living donors in 23 patients and in 80 from cadavers. Surprisingly, only 3 of the 103 Kaposi's sarcoma patients (3%) had more than one transplant, whereas in the rest of the series of cancer patients in whom the number of transplants is known, 262 of 2608 recipients (10%) had two or more transplants.

The immunosuppressive regimen of the Kaposi's sarcoma patients did not differ significantly from that of other transplant patients who developed de novo malignancies. All 103 had received corticosteroids, 93 azathioprine, 31 local radiotherapy to the graft, 25 antilymphocyte globulin, and 16 cyclosporine, 9 underwent splenectomy, 7 received actinomycin D, 3 cyclophosphamide, and 1 chlorambucil. In the entire series of 2817 tumors, Kaposi's sarcoma made up 16 of 162 (10%) of neoplasms in cyclosporine-treated patients compared with 87 of 2655 (3%) malignancies in patients given conventional immunosuppressive therapy.

Of the 103 patients, 7 (7%) had second primary malignancies. One patient each had been treated before transplantation for NHL, multiple myeloma, and carcinoma of the uterine cervix. After transplantation 2 patients developed lymphomas and 1 each developed a carcinoma of the colon and carcinoma of the thyroid gland.

Kaposi's sarcoma appeared a remarkably short time after transplantation, an average of 22 months (range 2–225.5). This contrasts with the other 2532 transplant patients whose cancers appeared an average of 60 months (range 1–253) after transplantation. In cyclosporine-treated patients, Kaposi's sarcoma appeared particularly early at an average of 10 (range 2–20.5) months.

Skin lesions were absent in 7 patients (7%). The occurrence of this neoplasm in the absence of skin manifestations is extremely rare (6,8). In the present series, 66 patients (64%) were classified as having "benign" Kaposi's sarcoma as they had lesions involving the skin and/or the oropharyngolaryngeal mucous membranes. Of these recipients, 5 had questionable internal visceral lesions but apparently these were not confirmed. The "malignant" variety of Kaposi's sarcoma with involvement of the internal organs was seen in 37 patients (36%). Whether this represents a high incidence is difficult to ascertain as the frequency of visceral involvement in classic Kaposi's sarcoma ranges from "about 10%" to 33% to a "high percentage" (6,8). The major sites of visceral involvement were the alimentary tract and lungs. Of the 37 patients, 7 (19%) had lymph node involvement.

Of the 66 patients with "benign" disease, 33 (50%) had complete remission following treatment. Most remissions followed local tumor excision or radiotherapy, sometimes combined with reduction of immunosuppressive therapy, and 5 patients received chemotherapy. Of great importance is that 8 remissions (24% of the remissions) occurred when the *only* treatment was drastic reduction or cessation of immunosuppressive therapy. Such treatment contributed to the remissions in several other patients as lesions started to regress after this change but before radiotherapy or chemotherapy or both were added. However, it must be emphasized that drastic reduction of immunosuppressive therapy was not followed invariably by regression of the lesions. In fact, in some cases the disease remained unchanged or even spread.

Of the 66 patients with "benign" Kaposi's sarcoma, 22 died. Most deaths (14) resulted from infection or from graft rejection and infection. One patient each died of a perforated peptic ulcer, perforation of the bowel, lymphoma, and anesthetic complications. In 3 patients the cause of death is unknown. In another patient an autopsy examination could not be obtained and the cause of death was listed as "possible complications of Kaposi's sarcoma." The average length of follow-up of the 66 patients from the time of diagnosis of Kaposi's sarcoma was 37 months (range 0.5–155).

Of the 37 patients with the "malignant" variety of Kaposi's sarcoma, 5 (14%) had complete remissions. These occurred following chemotherapy in 4 patients and radiotherapy in 1. In addition, immunosuppressive therapy was reduced or discontinued. Of the 37 patients, 25 died. In 22 cases Kaposi's sarcoma either caused the fatal outcome or contributed very significantly to it. The length of follow-up of the patients with the "malignant" form of Kaposi's sarcoma averaged 21 months (range 0.5–131).

In the overall series of 103 patients, 56 (54%) are currently alive. Almost half the deaths were from Kaposi's sarcoma.

Kaposi's sarcoma in transplant patients differs from that seen in AIDS in that lymph node involvement is rare, visceral disease is less common, and fatalities from Kaposi's sarcoma are less frequent. In addition, the immunosuppression in transplant patients can be reduced or totally stopped with the possibility of subsequent regression of the lesions (8), whereas in AIDS persistence of the immunodeficiency is a major feature (11,14).

OTHER IMMUNOSUPPRESSED PATIENTS

Immunosuppressive therapy is used to treat a variety of autoimmune diseases, chronic inflammatory disorders, and diseases of obscure etiology (7). In addition, immunosuppression may be an unwanted side effect of radiotherapy or chemotherapy used in the treatment of cancer, and paradoxically, second malignancies may develop as a consequence of such treatment (7). Penn (8) collected

35 cases [32 previously reported (8) and 3 recent cases (30–32)] of Kaposi's sarcoma from the literature that occurred after deliberate or unintentional immunosuppressive therapy. The patients represented an older group than those in the three categories already described; their ages ranged from 12 to 83 years (average 63). Males outnumbered females by 2:1. The predominant ethnic and racial groups, when stated, were Jewish (8 patients), Norwegian (7 patients), and Italian (6 patients). The most common underlying diseases that required treatment prior to the onset of Kaposi's sarcoma were other malignancies, mostly lymphomas (11 patients), pemphigus vulgaris or pemphigoid (9 patients), and rheumatoid arthritis (3 patients). When stated, the most common immunosuppressive therapies used were adrenal corticosteroids (26 patients), azathioprine (5 patients), and radiation therapy (5 patients). The average time of appearance of Kaposi's sarcoma after treatment was 41 months (range 1–228 months). In 10 patients (29%), visceral lesions (involving subcutaneous lymph nodes in 2 patients) were present, and in another patient the disease was described as "progressive." With the exception of 2 patients in whom the distribution of the lesions was not stated, all had skin involvement by Kaposi's sarcoma. In the overall series, 17 patients (49%) had other cancers in addition to Kaposi's sarcoma and 3 of these patients each had two additional neoplasms besides Kaposi's sarcoma.

There are several possible explanations for the development of these malignancies (8). One is that their appearance may have been quite coincidental. In some patients, not included with the 35 cases analyzed, Kaposi's sarcoma and a nonmalignant disease occurred more or less simultaneously. The two disorders either were completely unrelated or shared a common etiology. A second possibility is that Kaposi's sarcoma developed in the course of certain autoimmune, chronic inflammatory, and other nonmalignant diseases, which are themselves complicated by defects in immunity and an increased incidence of cancer (7,8). A third explanation is that Kaposi's sarcoma is frequently associated with other malignancies, particularly lymphomas. Lymphomas are frequently associated with defects in immunity that may have predisposed the patients to Kaposi's sarcoma (see Discussion). On the other hand, some investigators believe that Kaposi's sarcoma should be considered, along with leukemia and lymphoma, as part of a disease spectrum affecting the lymphoreticular system (5). In addition, it is possible that Kaposi's sarcoma and the various associated neoplasms had common etiopathogenic mechanisms (33). This possibility is mentioned further in the Discussion. A fourth possibility is that the immunosuppressive treatment per se caused the development of Kaposi's sarcoma. Unfortunately there are very few statistical data on the incidence of Kaposi's sarcoma in immunosuppressed nontransplant patients, and the cases analyzed in this section are derived mainly from isolated case reports. In the only study with statistical data, 7 of 49 Kaposi's sarcoma patients (14%), reported from Norway, had prior immunosuppressive therapy (34). However, the comparison population of 242 consecutive patients with basal cell carcinomas of the skin not treated with immunosuppressive therapy is not a satisfactory control as the patients were not matched for age, sex, and underlying disorders, many of which were autoimmune diseases.

DISCUSSION

The immunosuppressed state of AIDS patients with Kaposi's sarcoma has already been mentioned. Immunosuppression, as determined by depressed lymphocyte blastogenic responses to various mitogens in vitro, in vivo cutaneous anergy, or depressed immunoglobulin responses to various antigens, also has been described in classic Kaposi's sarcoma, in organ transplant recipients, and in African Kaposi's sarcoma (4,29,35–37). It has been suggested that chronic endemic malaria among Central African blacks may immunosuppress individuals and predispose them to infection by other agents, such as CMV, which may cause Kaposi's sarcoma in much the same way that chronic malaria and EBV are believed to cause African Burkitt's lymphoma (38). The demographic distribution of

Kaposi's sarcoma in Africa, however, does not support an etiologic relationship to malarial endemicity (3).

Two aspects of depressed immunity in Kaposi's sarcoma need to be considered. One is that an advanced malignancy per se may cause immunosuppression (7). This may explain the immunologic findings in some of the patients described here and is reinforced by the observation that patients with the benign localized form of Kaposi's sarcoma tend not to be anergic on repeated skin testing (35,36).

The other possibility is that depressed immunity plays an important role in the development of Kaposi's sarcoma. Several observations in favor of this possibility need to be discussed. First, Kaposi's sarcoma is frequently associated with other neoplasms (33). These tumors may precede or follow the appearance of Kaposi's sarcoma. In particular, lymphomas have been noted together with Kaposi's sarcoma in classic Kaposi's sarcoma (33), in AIDS patients (9,10), in immunosuppressed nontransplant patients (see above) (8), and in transplant patients (see above) (6–8). What is the significance of this association? Both types of cancer are accompanied by deficient cell-mediated immune responses (8, 35). It is conceivable that the one neoplasm could predispose to the other, or that some common factor may make patients susceptible to both tumors by causing immunosuppression or by some other mechanism (3,5). Further evidence in favor of an etiologic role of depressed immunity in Kaposi's sarcoma is that when immunosuppressive therapy was drastically reduced in several organ transplant recipients with the disease, complete regression occurred. In fact, 24% of all remissions of Kaposi's sarcoma in transplant patients with "benign" disease were produced in this way without any other form of treatment. The most telling evidence supporting an etiologic role of depressed immunity in Kaposi's sarcoma is that patients who received immunosuppressive therapy, or AIDS patients, had intense depression of immunity that *preceded* the appearance of the cancer by many weeks or months.

Two observations, however, do not favor depressed immunity as a cause of Kaposi's sarcoma. First, it is difficult to explain the paucity of Kaposi's sarcoma cases in a group of 14 congenital immunodeficiency diseases, such as the Wiskott-Aldrich syndrome and ataxia-telangiectasia (39), despite severe defects in cellular or humoral immunity or in both. One has no explanation for the high incidence of NHL in these profoundly immunodeficient patients compared with the rarity of Kaposi's sarcoma. Second, in a comprehensive study of cell-mediated and humoral immunity in endemic African Kaposi's sarcoma, Kestens et al. (40) were able to show no significant differences between patients and controls.

Depressed immunity may facilitate the development of Kaposi's sarcoma in several ways. The immune surveillance hypothesis (7,41,42) assigns an important role to the lymphoreticular system for the recognition and destruction of evolving neoplasms. It could be argued that if impaired immune surveillance were important one would expect an increased incidence of all types of cancer, not the disproportionately high incidence of Kaposi's sarcoma and NHL seen in immunosuppressed patients. However, it is possible that if immunosuppressed patients were to live long enough they might eventually develop epithelial cancers, which generally have long latent periods. Carcinomas of the breast, bronchus, prostate, and colon would then appear in proportions similar to those seen in the general population. Immunosuppressed patients tend to die at an earlier stage from intercurrent infections, Kaposi's sarcoma, and lymphomas (7).

Normally the extent of immune reactions is limited by cellular and humoral feedback mechanisms. If these are impaired there may be unrestrained proliferation of lymphocytes (7,43), which may evolve into lymphomas or Kaposi's sarcoma, which some workers believe to be tumors of lymphoreticular origin (3,9). The proliferating lymphocytes liberate various growth factors, including angiogenesis factor, which may stimulate lymphatic endothelial cells, already primed by a prior CMV infection, to undergo neoplastic proliferation (9). This theory is discussed in greater detail in Chapter 4.

In several experimental models, repeated or continuous administration of foreign antigens resulted in a high incidence of malignant lymphomas (7). Prolonged exposure to the foreign histocompatibility antigens of a transplanted organ, repeated infections by viruses, fungi, bacteria, and protozoa, or repeated exposure to antigens in allogeneic semen may perhaps explain the high incidence of Kaposi's sarcoma in the various groups of immunosuppressed patients described here (8).

Immunosuppression may favor the development of Kaposi's sarcoma in another way, namely, through activation of oncogenic viruses. An immunologic reaction, such as rejection of a transplanted organ, may activate latent endogenous oncornaviruses (44). The close resemblance of many aspects of Kaposi's sarcoma to murine sarcoma virus infection suggests a viral etiology (3). The frequent history of relapses and remissions of an individual nodule of Kaposi's sarcoma and the occasional history of apparently spontaneous cures of the "classic" variety of Kaposi's sarcoma is also in favor of an infective etiology (3). This possibility is strengthened by the short induction time of Kaposi's sarcoma after the onset of immunosuppression as seen in organ transplant and AIDS patients. Another point in favor of an infective etiology is the remissions of Kaposi's sarcoma in transplant patients when immunosuppressive therapy is drastically reduced (8), suggesting that the immune system is able to recover and to destroy the causative infectious agent and the cancer. Furthermore, the occurrence of clusters of the disease in endemic areas of Africa and among AIDS patients also favors involvement by an infectious agent. CMV has been most strongly implicated as a possible causative factor in Kaposi's sarcoma (5). CMV infections are very common in organ transplant and AIDS patients (7,45). CMV is a member of the herpes group of DNA viruses, numerous members of which have been linked to various forms of neoplasia (7). Not only may CMV by itself cause profound immunosuppression in humans (46), but it has also been shown to transform cells, including human cells (5,47). Epidemiologic, serologic, and virologic studies have linked CMV and Kaposi's sarcoma and are discussed in detail in Chapter 4.

Questions have been raised about a possible direct role of HIV in the etiology of Kaposi's sarcoma. However, seroepidemiologic studies of endemic African Kaposi's sarcoma have not shown any increased antibody titers to the virus (27). Furthermore, molecular hybridization of DNA obtained from Kaposi's sarcoma tumor tissue with cloned HIV genome failed to show evidence of virus infection (11).

Another factor that may contribute to the impaired immunity of AIDS patients and the development of Kaposi's sarcoma in homosexual men is the use of volatile nitrites as recreational drugs (16).These agents are profoundly immunosuppressive to human lymphocytes in vitro and may permit the expression of a potentionally oncogenic virus. Furthermore, their by-products are metabolized to N-nitroso compounds, which are highly carcinogenic in many animal species. In addition, they may cause dilatation of blood vessels in the rectal mucosa during anogenital intercourse, which could facilitate the entry of a transmissable viral agent or the passage of sperm.

Another theory that links immune disturbances and oncogenic viruses in the etiology of Kaposi's sarcoma is that of Warner and O'Loughlin (48). They postulate a chronic immunologic reaction between antigenically altered or transformed lymphoid cells and normal lymphocytes. In the course of this graft-versus-host type of activity, an angiogenesis factor is liberated and intense proliferation of mesenchymal and endothelial cells ensues. During this reaction an oncogenic virus is either transferred to or induced in the cells that are responding to the angiogenesis factor. This leads to neoplastic transformation of these cells in an environment that is conducive to the progressive growth of the virally transformed, vasoformative mesenchyme.

If immunosuppression and oncogenic viruses are important in the etiology of Kaposi's sarcoma, we may question why this neoplasm occurs only in a small percentage of people who may be at risk (8). Genetic factors may play a decisive role in determining which individuals are susceptible. These may explain the ethnic and racial distribution of Kaposi's sarcoma. The rarity of familial cases and lack of consanguinity are factors against simple Mendelian dominant or recessive inheritance but do not negate the possibility that there is a genetic predisposition to the disease.

Recently, more precise information on HLA-associated variations in genetic susceptibility has been obtained from studies of 39 patients with Kaposi's sarcoma, some with the classic form of the disease that affects older individuals and the remainder in homosexual patients with the aggressive variant of the disease (49). A significant increase in HLA-DR5 occurred in both groups. Decreases in HLA-B8 and HLA-DR3 and an increase in homozygosity for the Gm haplotype 3;5,13 were also noted. The results suggest that HLA and Gm-linked immune response factors are causally associated in the induction of both forms of the disease (49). However, it should be noted that the HLA-DR5 findings have not been confirmed in at least one study (50).

SUMMARY AND CONCLUSIONS

Kaposi's sarcoma has different clinical forms that may have different causes. Multiple factors probably play a role in the causation of any individual case of Kaposi's sarcoma. Of these, genetic predisposition and chronic immunosuppression appear to be of major importance. Repeated or continuous antigenic stimulation produced by organ allografts or chronic or repeated infections also appears to play a role. Heavy and persistent CMV infections, with frequent reactivations, may also be important. Only a small percentage of persons at risk develop Kaposi's sarcoma, probably because of genetic predisposition to the disease.

Intensive investigation of Kaposi's sarcoma in immunosuppressed patients may lead to an understanding of how impaired immunity contributes to the development of cancer; which genetic factors control the immune response; genetic susceptibility or resistance to cancer; and how viruses cause cancer in humans and animals. It is hoped that such work may lead to the discovery of better methods to restore impaired immunity and to the development of a vaccine or an effective antiviral agent against HIV infection. Such developments may relegate Kaposi's sarcoma to its original status as a medical curiosity.

ACKNOWLEDGMENTS

The author wishes to thank his many colleagues throughout the world who generously contributed data concerning their patients to the Cincinnati Transplant Tumor Registry. This chapter was supported in part by Grant Number 6985 from the Veterans Administration.

REFERENCES

1. Oettlé, AG. Geographical and racial differences in the frequency of Kaposi's sarcoma as evidence of environmental or genetic causes. Acta Union Int Contra Cancrum 1962; 18:330–63.
2. Rothman S. Remarks on sex, age, and racial distribution of Kaposi's sarcoma and on possible pathogenetic factors. Acta Union Int Contra Cancrum 1962; 18:326–9.
3. Templeton AC. Kaposi's sarcoma. In: Andrade R, Gumport SL, Popkin GL, Rees TD, eds. Cancer of the Skin: Biology, Diagnosis, Management. Vol 2. Philadelphia, WB Saunders, 1976:1183–225.
4. Harwood AR, Osaba D, Hofstader SL, Goldstein MB, Cardella CJ, Holecek MJ, Kunynetz R, Giammarco RA. Kaposi's sarcoma in recipients of renal transplants. Am J Med 1979; 67:759–65.
5. Safai B, Good RA. Kaposi's sarcoma: a review and recent developments. Ca 1981; 31:2–12.
6. Penn I. Kaposi's sarcoma in organ transplant recipients: report of 20 cases. Transplantation 1979; 27:8–11.
7. Penn I. The occurrence of cancer in immune deficiencies. Curr Prob Cancer 1982; 6:1–64.
8. Penn I. Kaposi's sarcoma in immunosuppressed patients. J Clin Lab Immunol 1983; 12:1–10.
9. Ziegler JL, Templeton AC, Vogel CL. Kaposi's sarcoma: a comparison of classical, endemic, and epidemic forms. Semin Oncol 1984; 11:47–52.
10. Ziegler JL, Levy JA. Acquired immunodeficiency syndrome and cancer. In: Klein G, ed. Advances in Viral Oncology. Vol 5. New York, Raven Press, 1985:239–55.

11. Fauci AS, Masur H, Gelmann EP, Markham PD, Hahn GH, Lane HC. The acquired immunodeficiency syndrome. Ann Intern Med 1985; 102:800–13.
12. Krigel RL. Prognostic factors in Kaposi's sarcoma. In: Friedman-Kien AE, Laubenstein LJ, eds. AIDS: The Epidemic of Kaposi's Sarcoma and Opportunistic Infections. New York, Masson Publishing, 1984.
13. Davies JNP, Lothe F. Kaposi's sarcoma in African children. Acta Union Int Contra Cancrum 1962; 18:394–9.
14. Gottlieb MS, Groopman JE, Weinstein WM, Fahey JL, Detels R. The acquired immunodeficiency syndrome. Ann Intern Med 1983; 99:208–20.
15. Shearer GM, Levy RB. Noninfectious cofactors in susceptibility to AIDS: possible contributions of semen, HLA alloantigens, and lack of natural resistance. Ann NY Acad Sci 1984; 437:49–57.
16. Newell GR, Adams SC, Mansell PWA, Hersh EM. Toxicity, immunosuppressive effects and carcinogenic potential of volatile nitrites: possible relationship to Kaposi's sarcoma. Pharmacotherapy 1984; 4:284–91.
17. Report of the Centers for Disease Control Task Force on Kaposi's sarcoma and opportunistic infections. Epidemiologic aspects of the current outbreak of Kaposi's sarcoma and opportunistic infections. N Engl J Med 1982; 306:248–52.
18. Jaffe HW, Choi K, Thomas PA, et al. National case-control study of Kaposi's sarcoma and *Pneumocystis carinii* pneumonia in homosexual men. Part 1. Epidemiologic results. Ann Intern Med 1983; 99:145–51.
19. Bayley AC, Downing RG, Cheinsong-Popov R, Tedder RS, Dalgleish AG, Weiss RA. HTLV-III serology distinguishes atypical and endemic Kaposi's sarcoma in Africa. Lancet 1985; 1:359–61.
20. Friedman-Kien AE, Laubenstein LJ, Rubinstein P, Buimovici-Klein E, Marmor M, Stahl R, Spigland I, Kim KS, Zolla-Pazner S. Disseminated Kaposi's sarcoma in homosexual men. Ann Intern Med 1982; 96:693–700.
21. Potter DA, Danforth DN Jr, Macher AM, Longo DL, Stewart L, Masur H. Evaluation of abdominal pain in the AIDS patient. Ann Surg 1984; 199:332–9.
22. Rose HS, Balthazar EJ, Megibow AJ, Horowitz L, Laubenstein LJ. Alimentary tract involvement in Kaposi's sarcoma: radiographic and

endoscopic findings in 25 homosexual men. Am J Roentgenol 1982; 139:661–6.
23. Real FX, Krown SE. Spontaneous regression of Kaposi's sarcoma in patients with AIDS (letter to the editor). N Engl J Med 1985; 313:1659.
24. Janier M, Vignon MD, Cottenot F. Spontaneously healing Kaposi's sarcoma in AIDS (letter to the editor). N Engl J Med 1985; 312: 1638–9.
25. Douglass MC, Cruz C, Pelachyk JM. Kaposi's sarcoma and immunosuppression. Curr Concepts Skin Disorders 1980; 1:7–16.
26. Bayley AC. Aggressive Kaposi's sarcoma in Zambia. Lancet 1984; 1:1318–20.
27. Biggar RJ, Melbye M, Kestems L, Sarngadharan MG, DeFeyter M, Blattner WA, Gallo RC, Gigase PL. Kaposi's sarcoma in Zaire is not associated with HTLV-III infection (letter to the editor). N Engl J Med 1984; 311:1051–2.
28. Downing RG, Elgin RP, Bayley AC. African Kaposi's sarcoma and AIDS. Lancet 1984; 1:478–80.
29. Hardy MA, Goldfarb P, Levine S, Dattner A, Muggia FM, Levitt S, Weinstein E. De novo Kaposi's sarcoma in renal transplantation. Case report and brief review. Cancer 1976; 38:144–8.
30. Caulet T, Hibon E, Roth A, Behart C, Tholon J-P, Dupuy D, Fandre M. Sarcome de Kaposi viscéral associé à un carcinome médullaire thyroïdien chez une enfant en très longue rémission de leucémie lymphoblastique. Nouv Presse Med 1977; 6:2673–6.
31. Bellelli A, Azzarito C, Salvarani C, Baricchi R, Portioli I. Sarcoma di Kaposi in corso di terapia cortisonica. Descrizione di un caso clinico. G Clin Med 1982; 63:614–21.
32. Guillet G, Chouvet B, Thivolet J, Perrot H. Traitements immunosuppresseurs et maladie de Kaposi. A propos de 2 observations. Ann Dermatol Venereol 1980; 107:907–10.
33. Safai B, Miké V, Giraldo G, Beth E, Good RA. Association of Kaposi's sarcoma with second primary malignancies. Possible etiopathogenic implications. Cancer 1980; 45:1472–9.
34. Klepp O, Dahl O, Stenwig JT. Association of Kaposi's sarcoma and prior immunosuppressive therapy. A 5-year material of Kaposi's sarcoma in Norway. Cancer 1978; 42:2626–30.
35. Master SP, Taylor JF, Kyalwazi SK, Ziegler JL. Immunological studies in Kaposi's sarcoma in Uganda. Br Med J 1970; 1:600–2.

36. Taylor JF, Ziegler JL. Delayed cutaneous hypersensitivity reactions in patients with Kaposi's sarcoma. Br J Cancer 1974; 30:312–8.
37. Dobozy A, Husz S, Hunyadi J, Berkó G, Simon N. Immune deficiencies and Kaposi's sarcoma (letter to the editor). Lancet 1973; 2:625.
38. Gange RW, Jones EW. Kaposi's sarcoma and immunosuppressive therapy: an appraisal. Clin Exp Dermatol 1978; 3:135–46.
39. Filipovich AH, Zerbe D, Spector BD, Kersey JH. Lymphomas in persons with naturally occurring immunodeficiency disorders. In: McGrath IT, O'Conor GT, Ramot B, eds. Pathogenesis of Leukemias and Lymphomas: Environmental Influences. New York, Raven Press, 1984:225–34.
40. Kestens L, Melbye M, Biggar RJ, Stevens WJ, Piot P, DeMuynck A, Taelman H, DeFeyter M, Paluku L, Gigase P. Endemic African Kaposi's sarcoma is not associated with immunodeficiency. Int J Cancer 1985; 36:49–54.
41. Thomas L. Discussion of Medawar PB. Reactions to homologous tissue antigens in relation to hypersensitivity. In: Lawrence HS, ed. Cellular and Humoral Aspects of the Hypersensitive States. New York, Paul Hoeber, 1959:529–32.
42. Burnet FM. Immunological surveillance in neoplasia. Transplant Rev 1971; 7:3–25.
43. Schwartz RS. Another look at immunologic surveillance. N Engl J Med 1975; 293:181–4.
44. Hirsch MS, Proffitt MR, Black PH. Autoimmunity, oncornaviruses and lymphomagenesis. Contemp Top Immunobiol 1977; 6:209–27.
45. Drew WL, Conant MA, Miner RC, Huang E-S, Ziegler JL, Groundwater JR, Gullett JH, Volberding P, Abrams DI, Mintz L. Cytomegalovirus and Kaposi's sarcoma in young homosexual men. Lancet 1982; 2:125–7.
46. Rinaldo CR Jr, Carney WP, Richter BS, Black PH, Hirsch MS. Mechanisms of immunosuppression in cytomegaloviral mononucleosis. J Infect Dis 1980; 141:488–95.
47. Geder L, Lausch R, O'Neill F, Rapp F. Oncogenic transformation of human embryo lung cells by human cytomegalovirus. Science 1976; 192:1134–7.
48. Warner TFCS, O'Loughlin S. Kaposi's sarcoma: a byproduct of tumor rejection. Lancet 1975; 2:687–9.
49. Pollack MS, Safai B, Myskowski PL, Gold JWM, Pandey J, Dupont B.

Frequencies of HLA and GM immunogenetic markers in Kaposi's sarcoma. Tissue Antigens 1983; 2:1–8.

50. Abrams D. Lymphoproliferative diseases and Kaposi's sarcoma in homosexual males. In: Purtilo DT, ed. Immune Deficiency and Cancer. Epstein-Barr Virus and Lymphoproliferative Malignancies. New York, Plenum Press, 1984:385–400.

6

Etiology: Angiogenesis

John L. Ziegler
Veterans Administration Medical Center
and University of California
San Francisco, California

This chapter addresses the pathogenesis of Kaposi's sarcoma in light of recent developments in the relationship among oncogenes, growth factors, and cancer. Since Kaposi's sarcoma is indisputably vasogenic in origin (see Chapter 3), it is logical to examine endothelial cell biology and angiogenesis for potential etiologic clues. Warner and O'Loughlin in 1975 first advanced the hypothesis that angiogenic factors caused endothelial proliferation in Kaposi's sarcoma. They also proposed that Kaposi's sarcoma may be "self-perpetuating" by producing its own angiogenic factor. They believed that the angiogenic factor stimulation was the result of a chronic immunologic reaction, such as that in graft-versus-host or tumor rejection reactions (1).

In order to pursue the hypothesis that angiogenic factors operate in the pathogenesis of Kaposi's sarcoma, I review briefly some relevant background material. Students of oncogenesis have long sought a "final common pathway" by which varied environmental (e.g., chemicals or radiation) or genetic (e.g., viruses or heredity) perturbations lead to cancer. The oncogene hypothesis first advanced by Huebner and Todaro and redefined by Bishop has opened new avenues of research (2). Experiments in the areas of embryogenesis, tissue regeneration, atherogenesis, wound healing, and tumor-induced angiogenesis have revealed a complex array of biologic substances that regulate capillary growth. From this review I highlight the data supporting a hypothesis that links angiogenesis and Kaposi's sarcoma.

ONCOGENES

It has long been hypothesized that the neoplastic process occurs in a stepwise fashion and that the primary cause is alteration of DNA, which results in cell proliferation and transformation to the malignant state. The recent discovery of "oncogenes," highly conserved sets of cellular genes that govern cell growth and differentiation, has greatly advanced research into the molecular genetics of the neoplastic process (2–5). Simply put, oncogenes or "proto-oncogenes" (i.e., constitutively inactive genes) are genetic sequences that are normally dormant but become active during embryogenesis, in response to injury, or in the regulation of replicating tissues.

Under normal circumstances these gene families, which undoubtedly act in concert, direct cell growth and differentiation in an orderly fashion. However, when disrupted by any of a variety of insults, these genes may become constitutively or quantitatively altered such that their protein products are abnormal in configuration or are overproduced, leading the cell to an autonomous proliferative state. A corollary to this hypothesis is the existence of a family of "antioncogenes" that exert negative regulatory effects on gene expression at the level of RNA transcription (6).

The last decade of research has disclosed over 40 different oncogenes of viral or cellular origin. These have been grouped into two broad categories: genes whose products (e.g., *c-myc*) affect the cell nucleus and "immortalize" the cell; and genes whose products (e.g., *c-ras*) affect the cell cytoplasm and confer anchorage-independent growth (5). The mechanisms of oncogene activation can also be generalized: nuclear-acting genes become "deregulated" by chromosomal translocation or other genomic perturbations that permit them to become expressed; cytoplasm-acting genes become activated largely by point mutational events (Table 1).

Table 1 Activation and Functions of Proto-oncogenes

	Site of action of gene product	
	Nucleus	Cytoplasm
Prototype oncogene	*myc*	*ras*
Mechanism of activation	Deregulation	Mutation
Function	Transactivation	Growth factors; growth factor receptors; post-receptor signals
Effect on cell	Immortalization	Anchorage; independence

Source: From Reference 5.

The phenotypic consequences of the overexpressed or abnormal oncogene products are largely speculative. Generally speaking, nuclear-acting gene products alter the ability of the cell to respond to normal regulatory signals. Cytoplasmic oncogene products may affect cell regulatory processes that lead to production of growth factors, expression of growth factor receptors, or stimulation of "second messenger" signals of cell proliferation. Cancer appears to be the end stage of a multistep process that evolves over long periods of time, involves the interactions of several families of oncogenes, and is strongly influenced by microenvironmental factors (e.g., immunologic, hormonal, and vascular). Experimentally, the process has been divided into "initiation" (alteration of gene structure) and "promotion" (altered gene expression) phases. Once formed, a tumor continues to evolve and adapt phenotypically to the host and becomes increasingly heterogeneous. This adds a third phase to tumorigenesis, "progression." A role for oncogenes in this clonal metamorphosis has been postulated (7).

In 1980, Sporn and Todaro proposed that some neoplasms are self-perpetuating by means of the autonomous production of "autocrine" transforming growth factors (TGF) and TGF receptors (8). Already there was a list of polypeptide growth factors that act by endocrine (distant cell targets), paracrine (local cell targets), or autocrine (same target cell) mechanisms (9).

THE ENDOTHELIAL CELL

The endothelium comprises a monocellular lining of all vessels: arteries, arterioles, capillaries, venules and veins of the systemic circulation; and the lymphatic vasculature. Endothelial cells perform a variety of vital functions that includes production of stromal collagen and fibronectin, delivery of oxygen and nutrients to tissues, removal of waste products, maintenance of hemostasis, responsiveness to injury and inflammation, participation in circulatory homeostasis, and specialized functions, for example in the choroid plexus, renal glomerulus, corpus luteum, and retina. Endothelial cells are remarkably versatile, pluripotent mesenchymal cells that respond adaptively to the functional demands of their environment (10).

Studies of wound healing and early solid tumor growth describe several stages of neoangiogenesis: endothelial cells migrate through the vessel wall by proteolytic degradation of the basement membrane; a capillary sprout is formed in alignment with the angiogenic stimulus and a lumen is formed; the sprouts join to form a capillary loop; new sprouts eventually form an entire capillary network, and the stroma (basement membrane and pericytes) is formed (11,12). Early in this process the capillary bed is fragile, giving rise to the easy bleeding encountered in granulation tissue and tumors.

ANGIOGENIC FACTORS

Much of the progress in angiogenesis was prompted by a search for factors that would promote wound healing, on one hand, and for "antiangiogenesis" factors that would retard cancer growth on the other. Research was accelerated by the development of sensitive in vitro assays of angiogenesis using the rabbit cornea, hamster cheek pouch, and chick allantoic membrane. These bioassays detected a number of substances that stimulate angiogenesis (13).

Angiogenic factors can now be divided into two groups: (1) agents that influence the migration of endothelial cells, and (2) polypeptide growth factors that affect proliferation and differentiation of endothelial cells (11,14). The variety of biologically active angiogenic factors has led to the "cascade hypothesis" whereby various substances influence angiogenesis either independently or by synergistic mechanisms (11). Some endothelial growth factors exert paradoxical effects in various bioassays, indicating that neovascularization is a highly complex, homeostatic process.

Table 2 displays several cofactors that influence angiogenesis. The angiogenic effect of heparin may be explained by its molecular affinity to several polypeptide endothelial cell growth factors. The

Table 2 Angiogenic Cofactors

Factor	Mechanism of action	References
Heparin	Binds and stabilizes endothelial growth factors	15–17
Hyaluronic acid	Disrupts extracellular matrix	18
Prostaglandin E	Chemotaxis of endothelial cells	19, 20
Copper	Chemotaxis of endothelial cells	19
Temperature, pH, O_2 tension, lactate	Binding of growth factors and endothelial response	9–11

glycosaminoglycan carbohydrate may act to stabilize the tertiary structure of the polypeptide, conferring heat and acid stability and facilitating its interaction with growth factor receptors on the endothelial cell (15,16). Heparin affinity has been exploited as a means of chromatographic separation of growth factors from various tissues (17).

Another angiogenesis cofactor, hyaluronic acid, is postulated to assist endothelial migration into wounds (18). Prostaglandins of the E series and copper ions also stimulate angiogenesis by unknown mechanisms (19,20). Finally, microenvironmental factors, such as pH, temperature, lactate concentration, and oxygen tension, influence endothelial cell migration and proliferation (9–11,21).

Polypeptide endothelial cell growth factors (ECGF) are broadly subdivided into primary and secondary mitogens (11). The primary ECGF fall into two biochemical categories: anionic (acidic) and cationic (basic). Nomenclature for various growth factors that cause endothelial proliferation is not standardized; until all putative factors are fully characterized and classified, the nosology of ECGF will remain confused (17).

Evidence thus far reveals two distinct families of heparin-binding ECGF that are structurally related and share varying degrees of functional homology (22–25). Gospodarowicz and colleagues have isolated and characterized acidic and basic forms of fibroblast growth factor (FGF). These two forms have a high degree of homology and, although localized to chromosomes number 5 and 4, respectively, are thought to derive from a common ancestral gene (17). They believe that the many endothelial growth factors will ultimately be found to be related structurally to acidic or basic FGF. Basic FGF displays highly potent mitogenic activity of endothelial and other mesodermal cells. It also exhibits differentiating effects and modulates the production of components of the extracellular matrix. Acidic FGF has thus far been isolated only from brain and retina and is 30- to 100-fold less potent than basic FGF. Both factors exhibit weak homology with interleukin-1 and certain neuropeptides (17). Figure 1 displays the variety of endothelial growth factors related to acidic and basic FGF (17).

Angiogenin, a tumor-derived ECGF, has potent angiochemotactic properties and has been recently isolated, genetically cloned, and sequenced (26). Secondary factors that exhibit endothelial mitogenic activity, such as epidermal growth factor, platelet-derived growth factor, insulin, transferrin, and interleukin-1, may not play important roles in angiogenesis (11).

Recently, another family of polypeptide angiogenic factors has been characterized: the transforming growth factors (TGF) α and β (13,27). TGF-α shares 35% homology with epidermal growth factor and is synthesized by many normal and malignant tissues. It is a postulated mediator of autocrine growth regulation and may play a role in the neovascularization of solid tumors.

TGF-β also exerts local angiogenic activity when injected into newborn mice, but the mechanism of action is uncertain since in vitro TGF-β inhibits DNA synthesis in endothelial cells (27,28). A possible explanation for this apparent paradox is that TGF-β induces angiogenesis in vivo by secondary mechanisms, causing endothelial migration via chemotactic factors or inducing production of other angiogenic factors in the microenvironment (28). It is now clear that both TGF-α and TGF-β are fundamental regulatory molecules that act by autocrine and paracrine mechanisms (29).

Abundant factors elaborated during immune and inflammatory

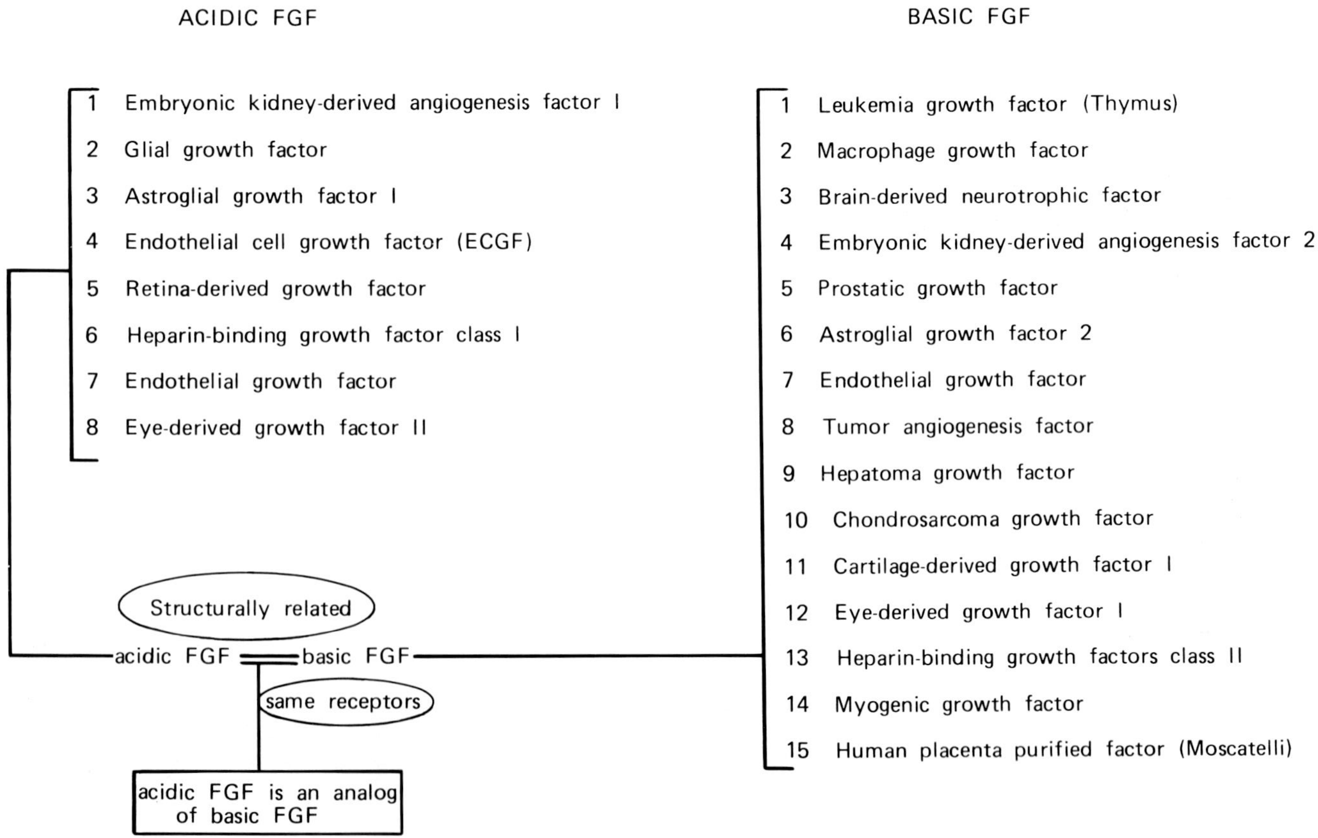

Figure 1 Nomenclature of various endothelial growth factors reported in the literature. (Reproduced by kind permission of D. Gospodarowicz, Reference 56).

responses stimulate angiogenesis. Some of these mediate the migration of endothelial cells, others affect endothelial cell proliferation and differentiation, and still others influence the formation of neovascular stroma. Studies of inflammatory cells and platelets have yielded additional angiogenic factors.

Supernatants from mixed leukocyte cultures stimulate endothelial cell proliferation and yield a crude endothelial mitogenic lymphokine called ECL-1 (30). ECL-1 is produced by T lymphocytes, is distinct from the interleukins, and does not bind to heparin. Its relationship to other angiogenic growth factors is under study. Macrophages also produce a variety of angiogenic factors, including FGF (17,31,32).

ENDOTHELIAL CELLS AND THE IMMUNE SYSTEM

In order to draw inferences regarding the pathogenesis of Kaposi's sarcoma in patients with the acquired immunodeficiency syndrome (AIDS), I shall consider briefly the structural and functional interactions between endothelium and the immune system. The lymphatic endothelium functions primarily as a cephalad drainage system for extracellular fluid. The lymphatic circulation also provides interconnections within and between lymph nodes and a transportation mode for triglycerides absorbed from the gut (33). In addition to a rich capsular lymphatic network, lymph nodes are well vascularized by an afferent and efferent vascular bed that enters and exits at the hilum. These lymphatic and capillary vessels also receive autonomic enervation.

Endothelial cells play an important role in lymphocyte traffic. Receptors on "high endothelial venules" in lymph nodes and Peyer's patches bind to specific ligands on T and B lymphocytes and influence the localization of lymphocyte subsets in lymph nodes (34) and in inflamed tissues (35). In addition to monitoring lymphocyte traffic, endothelial cells participate in the immune response, acting as antigen-presenting cells (36). Because of their surface expression of class II histocompatibility antigens, endothelial cells may be the targets of graft rejection reactions (37).

Certain pathologic conditions give rise to excessive angiogenic activity in lymphoid tissue. As a group, these conditions have been called angiolymphoproliferative syndromes (38). The best characterized are the syndromes of angioimmunoblastic lymphadenopathy (AILD) and Castleman's disease (39,40). AILD often follows viral infection and is thought to be a result of excessive T-cell effects on B cells (39). Regrettably, there are no studies of AILD that have examined the pathogenesis of vascular proliferation. Likewise, the angiofollicular proliferation in Castleman's disease is related to T-cell abnormalities but the relationship to angiogenesis is unknown (40). Finally, angiogenic lymphokines have been detected in lymph draining ischemic kidneys in the rat (41). Thus, although angiolymphoproliferative syndromes are well-described, the existance of angiogenic lymphokines from dysregulated lymphoid tissue can only be inferred (38).

In view of this, it is of considerable interest that Kaposi's sarcoma in lymph nodes from 6 AIDS patients was accompanied by "hypervascular follicular hyperplasia," a finding that was not observed in 10 AIDS patients without Kaposi's sarcoma (42). In addition, AILD was described in 2 patients with AIDS (43). Clearly, the lymphoproliferative immune response to HIV infection will induce, in some patients, an exaggerated angiogenic response in the affected lymph node. Further, the association of Kaposi's sarcoma with lymphoproliferative malignancies is well known (44). It seems logical to propose that angiogenic lymphokines are involved in the pathogenesis of Kaposi's sarcoma.

HYPOTHESIS: KAPOSI'S SARCOMA IS AN ENDOTHELIAL NEOPLASM PROVOKED BY LOCAL ANGIOGENIC FACTORS

As discussed by other authors in this book, the pathogenesis of Kaposi's sarcoma is multifactorial. I propose that one of the critical factors is the production, either paracrine or autocrine, of angiogenic growth factors (45,46). As discussed earlier, perturbation of the regulatory machinery that governs cell growth and differentiation leads to the stepwise progression to neoplasia. Kaposi's sarcoma in its earliest stages is not considered a neoplasm (47), but the tumor does evolve into a more anaplastic state in which many mesenchynal elements can be recognized (see Chapter 2). Angiogenic factors are likely to participate in the earliest stages of Kaposi's sarcoma and are perhaps involved in an autocrine manner as the neoplasm progresses.

Figure 2 outlines the dynamics of this hypothesis in patients with AIDS. The earliest event following infection with human immunodeficiency virus (HIV) is pronounced lymphoproliferation. Angiogenic lymphokines provoke local capillary and lymphatic endothelial cell hyperplasia. As discussed in Chapter 1, this propensity may have genetic determinants, as neoangiogenesis is prominent in patients with Kaposi's sarcoma and absent in controls (42). In some proliferating endothelial cells additional cofactors, such as activation of *c-sis* (48) or another transforming oncogene (49), confer further growth autonomy. As discussed earlier, basic FGF is a potent endothelial mitogen and activates both *c-myc* and *c-fos* oncogenes (17). Growing endothelial cells are also subject to normal regulatory restraints exerted in the microenvironment, and some proliferative lesions may differentiate, remain stable, or regress (Kaposi's sarcoma is prone to regress spontaneously). The exact nature and sequence of the transforming events (such as cytomegalovirus infection, circulating carcinogens, or evasion from immunologic surveillance) are speculative and are discussed in more detail in Chapters 1, 4, and 5.

If angiogenic growth factors play a primary role in the pathogenesis of Kaposi's sarcoma, then measures to counter this process have potential therapeutic value. One must assume the existence of natural inhibitors of angiogenesis that oppose or assist in the regulation of neovascularization (11–13,37). Many investigators have sought such antiangiogenesis factors in an effort to reduce the blood supply to tumors (12). An impressive list of such factors has

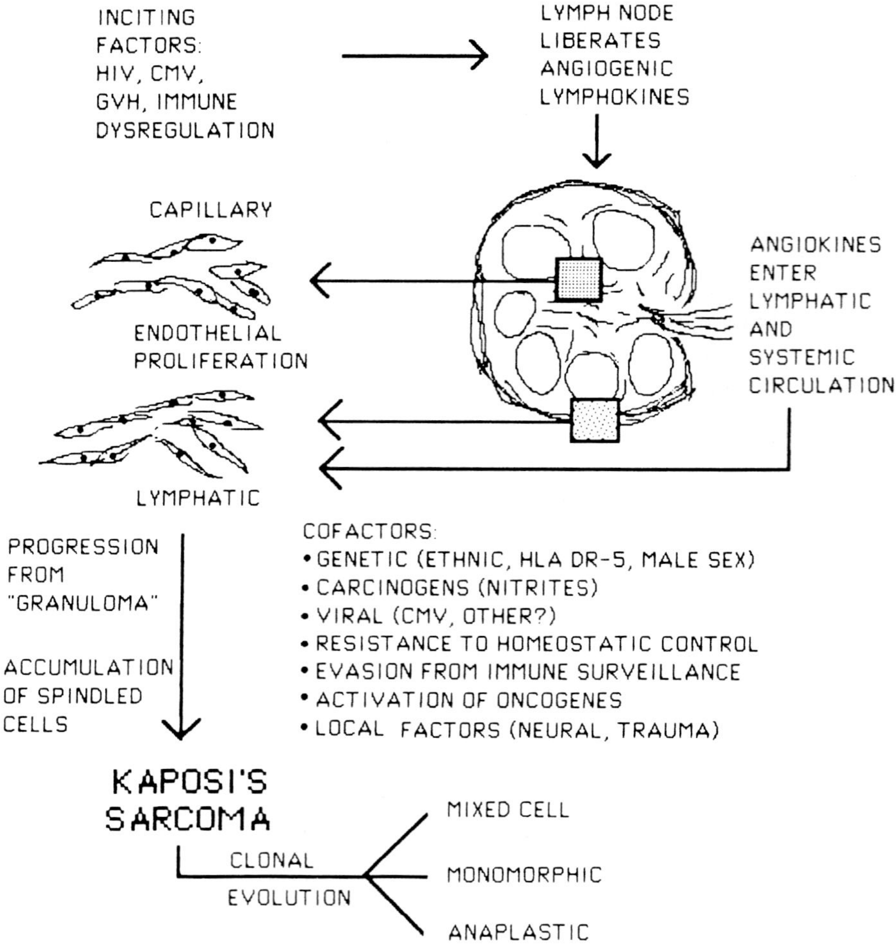

Figure 2 Role of angiogenesis factors in Kaposi's sarcoma. A variety of inciting factors perturb lymphocytes and macrophages that liberate abundant angiokines in a genetically susceptible host. Focal vascular proliferations (both lymphatic and capillary), both in lymph nodes and elsewhere, develop and progress under the influence of various cofactors into typical Kaposi's sarcoma lesions. Further clonal evolution confers a more malignant phenotype to account for the progressive clinical variants of tumor appearance and behavior.

accumulated. Because heparin binds ECGF, the heparin antagonist, protamine, inhibits angiogenesis (50). Shark cartilage extract, interferons, tumor necrosis factor, and TGF-β are some biologic materials that inhibit angiogenesis (51–53). A novel class of "angiostatic" steroids, acting in concert with heparin fragments, also inhibits angiogenesis (54). Finally, the use of monoclonal antibodies directed at the functional domain of angiogenic growth factors or their receptors has antiangiogenic potential (55). Although much has yet to be learned about the regulatory controls of angiogenesis, exploration of this process should yield considerable insight into oncogenesis and control of the neoplastic process (56). Kaposi's sarcoma provides an unusual paradigm for this avenue of research.

ACKNOWLEDGMENTS

The author wishes to thank Doctors Thomas Hunt and Denis Gospodarowicz for their helpful criticism in the preparation of this chapter.

RECENT DEVELOPMENTS

A role for angiogenesis in Kaposi's sarcoma is supported by several recent findings. A potent growth factor for Kaposi's sarcoma in tissue culture was derived from lymphocytes infected by human T cell lymphotropic virus type II (HTLV-II). The factor appears to be different from fibroblast growth factor (57). Thus, a lymphokine from a retrovirus-infected cell can stimulate growth of Kaposi's sarcoma. In a review of angiogenesis factors, Folkman and Klagsburn summarize the evidence for physiologic regulation of blood vessel growth (58). They postulate the existence of circulating angiogenesis inhibitors that possibly operate differently in women and men. Thus, the predominance of Kaposi's sarcoma in men may result from the appearance of a stimulating growth factor that overcomes physiologic restraints.

REFERENCES

1. Warner TFCS, O'Loughlin S. Kaposi's sarcoma. A byproduct of tumor rejection. Lancet 1975; 2:687–9.
2. Bishop JM. The molecular genetics of cancer. Nature 1986; 235: 305–11.
3. Weiss RA, Marshall CJ. Oncogenes. Lancet 1984; 2:1138–42.
4. Klein G, Klein E. Evolution of tumors and the impact of molecular oncology. Nature 1985; 315:190–5.
5. Weinberg RA. The action of oncogenes in the cytoplasm and nucleus. Science 1985; 230:770–6.
6. Green AR, Wyke JA. Antioncogenes. A subset of regulatory genes involved in carcinogenesis? Lancet 1985; 2:475–7.
7. Editorial. Molecular mechanisms of tumor evolution. Lancet 1986; 1:780–1.
8. Sporn MB, Todaro GT. Autocrine secretion and malignant transformation of cells. N Engl J Med 1980; 303:878–80.
9. Golde DW, Hershmann HR, Lusis AJ, Groopman JE. Growth factors. Ann Intern Med 1980; 92:650–62.
10. Thilo-Korner DGS, Freshney RI, eds. The Endothelial Cell: A Pluripotent Control Cell of the Vessel Wall. Basel, S Karger, 1982.
11. Maciag T. Angiogenesis. Prog Thromb Hemost 1984; 7:167–82.
12. Folkman J. How is blood vessel growth regulated in normal and neoplastic tissue? GHA Clowes Memorial Award Lecture. Cancer Res 1986; 46:467–73.
13. Folkman J. Toward an understanding of angiogenesis: search and discovery. Perspect Biol Med 1985; 29:10–36.
14. Schreiber AB, Winkler ME, Derynck R. Transforming growth factor—alpha: a more potent angiogenic mediator than epidermal growth factor. Science 1986; 232:1250–3.
15. Shing Y, Folkman J, Sullivan R, Butterfield C, Murray J, Kagsburn B. Heparin affinity: purification of tumor-derived capillary endothelial cell growth factor. Science 1984; 223:1296–9.
16. Maciag T, Mehlman T, Friesel R, Schrieber AB. Heparin binds endothelial cell growth factor, the principal endothelial cell mitogen in bovine brain. Science 1984; 225:932–5.
17. Gospodarowicz D, Neufeld G, Schweigerer, L. Review. Fibroblast growth factor. Mol Cell Endocrinol 1986; 46:187–204.
18. West DC, Hampson IN, Arnold F, Kumar S. Angiogenesis induced

by degradation products of hyaluronic acid. Science 1985; 228:324–6.

19. Ziche M, Jones J, Gullino PM. Role of prostaglandin E and copper in angiogenesis. JNCI 1982; 69:475–82.
20. Form DM, Auerbach R. PGE2 and angiogenesis. Proc Soc Exp Biol Med 1983; 172:214–8.
21. Jensen, JA, Hunt TK, Schevenstuhl H, Banda MJ. Effect of lactate, pyruvate, and pH on secretion of angiogenesis and mitogenesis factors by macrophages. Lab Invest 1986; 54:574–8.
22. Burgess WH, Mehlman T, Friesel R, Johnson WV, Maciag T. Multiple forms of endothelial cell growth factor. J Biol Chem 1985; 260:11389–92.
23. Jaye M, Howk R, Burgess W, et al. Human endothelial cell growth factor: cloning, nucleotide sequence, and chromosome localization. Science 1986; 233:541–5.
24. Abraham JA, Mergia A, Whang JL, et al. Nucleotide sequence of a bovine clone in coding the angiogenic protein, basic fibroblast growth factor. Science 1986; 233:545–8.
25. Shreiber AB, Kenney J, Kowalsky J, et al. A unique family of endothelial polypeptide mitogens: the antigenic and receptor cross-reactivity of bovine endothelial cell growth factor, brain-derived acidic fibroblast growth factor, and eye-derived growth factor-II. J Cell Biol 1985; 101:1623–26.
26. Fett JW, Strydom DJ, Lobb RR, et al. Isolation and characterization of angiogenin, an angiogenic protein from human carcinoma cells. Biochemistry 1985; 24:5480–6.
27. Roberts AB, Sporn MB, Assoian RF, et al. Transforming growth factor type β: rapid induction of fibrosis and angiogenesis in vivo and stimulation of collagen formation in vitro. Proc Natl Acad Sci USA 1986; 83:4167–71.
28. Hermark RL, Twardzik DR, Schwartz SM. Inhibition of endothelial regeneration by type-beta transforming growth factor from platelets. Science 1986; 233:1078–80.
29. Sporn MB, Roberts AB, Wakefield LM, Assoian RK. Transforming growth factor-β: biological function and chemical structure. Science 1986; 233:523–4.
30. Watt SL, Auerbach R. A mutagenic factor for endothelial cells obtained from mouse secondary mixed leukocyte cultures. J Immunol 1986; 136:197–202.

31. Polverini PJ, Cotran RS, Gimbrone MA, Unanue ER. Activated macrophages induce vascular proliferation. Nature 1977; 269:804–6.
32. Knighton DR, Hunt TK, Schenenstull H, Halliday BJ, Werb Z, Banda MJ. Oxygen tension regulates expression of angiogenesis factor by macrophages. Science 1983; 221:1283–5.
33. Weiss L. Histology. Cell and Tissue Biology. New York, Elsevier Biomedical, 1985:377.
34. Rosen SD, Singer MS, Yarnock TA, Stoolman LM. Involvement of sialic acid on endothelial cells in organ-specific lymphoid recirculation. Science 1985; 228:1005–8.
35. Jalkanen S, Steere AC, Fox RI, Butcher EC. A distinct endothelial cell recognition system that controls lymphocyte traffic into inflamed synovium. Science 1986; 233:556–8.
36. Pober JS, Collins T, Gimbrone MA, et al. Lymphocytes recognize human vascular endothelial and dermal fibroblast Ia antigens induced by recombinant interferon. Nature 1983; 305:726–9.
37. de Wall RMW, Bogman MJJ, Maass CN, Cornelissen LMH, Tax WJM, Koene RAP. Variable expression of Ia antigens on the vascular endothelium of mouse skin allografts. Nature 1983; 302:425–9.
38. DeCarvalho S. Angiokines, angiogenesis and angiolymphoproliferative syndromes (ALPS). Angiology 1983; 34:231–43.
39. Honda M, Smith HR, Steinberg AD. Studies of the pathogenesis of angioimmunoblastic lymphadenopathy. J Clin Invest 1985; 76:332–40.
40. Lachant NA, Sun NCJ, Leong LA, Oseao RS, Prince HE. Multicentric angiofollicular lymph node hyperplasia (Castleman's disease) followed by Kaposi's sarcoma in two homosexual males with the acquired immunodeficiency syndrome. J Clin Pathol 1985; 83:27–33.
41. Hollenberg NK, Paskins-Hurlburt AJ, Abrams HL. Collateral arterial formation. Lymph draining ischemic kidneys contain a neovascular stimulating agent of high molecular weight. Invest Radiol 1985; 20:58–61.
42. Harris NL. Hypervascular follicular hyperplasia and Kaposi's sarcoma in patients at risk for AIDS. N Engl J Med 1984; 310:462–3.
43. Blumenfeld W, Beckstead JA. Angioimmunoblastic lymphadenopathy with dysproteinemia (AILD) in homosexual males with the

acquired immunodeficiency syndrome (AIDS). Arch Pathol Lab Med 1983; 107:567–9.
44. Ullbright TM, Santa Cruz DJ. Kaposi's sarcoma. Relationship with hematologic, lymphoid, and thymic neoplasia. Cancer 1981; 47: 963–73.
45. Levy JA, Ziegler JL. Hypothesis. Acquired immunodeficiency syndrome is an opportunistic infection and Kaposi's sarcoma results from secondary immune stimulation. Lancet 1983; 2:78–81.
46. Ziegler JL, Templeton AC, Vogel CL. Kaposi's sarcoma: a comparison of classical, endemic and epidemic forms. Semin Oncol 1984; 11:47–52.
47. Costa J, Robson AL. Generalized Kaposi's sarcoma is not a neoplasm. Lancet 1983; 1:58.
48. Jaye M, McConathy E, Drohan W, Tong B, Devel T, Maciag T. Modulation of the *sis* gene transcript during endothelial cell differentiation in vitro. Science 1985; 228:882–4.
49. Lo S-C, Liotta LA. Vascular tumors produced by NIH 3T3 cells transfected with human AIDS Kaposi's sarcoma DNA. Am J Pathol 1985; 118:7–13.
50. Taylor S, Folkman J. Protamine is an inhibitor of angiogenesis. Nature 1982; 297:307–12.
51. Lee A, Langen R. Shark cartilage contains inhibitors of angiogenesis. Science 1983; 221:1185–7.
52. Editorial. Growth factors and malignancy. Lancet 1980; 2:317–8.
53. Cohen MC, Piccrano PT, Douglas WJ, et al. Migration inhibition of endothelial cells by lymphokine-containing supernatants. Science 1982; 215:301–2.
54. Crum R, Szabo S, Folkman J. A new class of steroids inhibits angiogenesis in the presence of heparin or a heparin fragment. Science 1985; 230:1375–7.
55. Shahabuddin S, Kumar S, West D, Arnold F. A study of angiogenesis factors from five different sources using a radioimmunoassay. Int J Cancer 1985; 35:87–91.
56. Gospodarowicz D, Neufeld G, Schweigerer L. Review. Molecular and biological characterization of fibroblast growth factor, an angiogenic factor which also controls the proliferation and differentiation of mesoderm and neuroectoderm derived cells. Cell Differ 1986; 19:1–17.

57. Nakamura S, Ensoli B, Salahuddin SZ, Biberfeld P, Gallo RC. Human T lymphotropic virus II (HTLV-II)-transformed cell lines release a potent growth factor for Kaposi's sarcoma (KS) cell lines. Clin Res 1987; 35:616A (abstract).
58. Folkman J, Klagsburn M. Angiogenic factors. Science 1987; 235:442–7.

7

Clinical Features and Staging

Paul A. Volberding
University of California
and San Francisco General Hospital
San Francisco, California

Kaposi's sarcoma is not a new disease, but in the setting of the acquired immunodeficiency syndrome (AIDS), this tumor has taken on many unique clinical features that make its management a challenge. Kaposi's sarcoma in AIDS has a broad clinical variation, the reasons for which are not well understood, and approaches to a uniform staging system remain tentative. This chapter reviews some aspects of the clinical presentation of Kaposi's sarcoma in AIDS patients, contrasting the tumor in this situation with its appearance in other clinical settings. I also review the current status of staging systems for Kaposi's sarcoma, recommending future efforts that will be required.

Kaposi's sarcoma was first recognized and described in the late 1800s by the noted Hungarian physician, Moritz Kaposi (1). The tumor he described afflicted elderly men and remained localized to the skin for much of its indolent clinical course. This variant of Kaposi's sarcoma, now often called classic Kaposi's sarcoma, was until recently the most frequent type seen in the United States.

In the early 1960s, a second population with a significant risk for Kaposi's sarcoma was reported in Central Africa. There, it was discovered that Kaposi's sarcoma was a common human malignancy—the most common cancer in some countries—and that it assumed, in some cases, clinical variants not previously described. In children, for example, Kaposi's sarcoma in Africa often appeared to be a much more aggressive cancer and one affecting the lymphatic system and visceral organs more frequently than the skin.

The third group affected by Kaposi's sarcoma outside of the current epidemic are patients iatrogenically immunosuppressed in the course of renal transplantation or in the treatment of a variety of autoimmune disorders. In this setting, Kaposi's sarcoma is often widespread and rapidly progressive, features shared by AIDS patients with this tumor.

CLINICAL PATHOLOGICAL CLASSIFICATION

Several variants of Kaposi's sarcoma have been described recognized by the gross appearance of malignant tumors. These variants of Kaposi's sarcoma, nodular, florid-infiltrative, and lymphadenopathic, are seen in differing proportions in all groups of patients affected by this malignancy whether related to AIDS or not (Table 1).

Nodular Kaposi's sarcoma, as the name implies, is characterized by cutaneous nodular lesions that vary in size from several millimeters to several centimeters in diameter (2–4) [Figures 1A,B (see Plate I, facing p. 178)]. These lesions are pigmented and because of the vascular nature of Kaposi's sarcoma, appear red to blue; however, some deeper lesions may be unpigmented. The early lesions of nodular Kaposi's sarcoma may be confused with common nonmalignant cutaneous disorders, including dermatofibromas. In Kaposi's sarcoma, cutaneous nodules are nonpruritic and usually not painful, although discomfort can be experienced, especially in dependent regions as tumor nodules enlarge. Nodular Kaposi's sarcoma does not usually cause necrosis of overlying normal skin and rarely invades underlying bony structures. Nodules of Kaposi's sarcoma in most clinical forms of the tumor can be seen on any part of the body but often tend to concentrate on the distal lower extremities. Nodular Kaposi's sarcoma is often the most indolent variant, except as will be described, in the AIDS setting.

Florid or *infiltrating* Kaposi's sarcoma represents a distinct second clinical form (2–4). Florid Kaposi's sarcoma lesions are frequent in African patients, are usually present in small numbers, but are large and exophytic [Figure 2 (see Plate I, facing p. 178)]. Necrosis of the surface of this tumor is common, and invasion of underlying bone and infiltration of adjacent normal structures are frequent. Although any part of the body may be affected by florid Kaposi's sarcoma, distal upper and lower extremity lesions are most common.

The third form of Kaposi's sarcoma seen primarily in African children is *lymphadenopathic* (2–6). Lymphadenopathic Kaposi's sarcoma primarily affects the lymphatic structures, particularly peripheral lymph nodes, often leaving the skin unaffected. Lymphadenopathic Kaposi's sarcoma typically has a rapidly progressive clinical course with a more rapid mortality than in most other Kaposi's sarcoma patients without AIDS.

Table 1 Clinical Variants of Kaposi's Sarcoma

Type	Ages	Lesion size (cm)	Distribution	Number	Superficial necrosis	Deep tissue invasion	Clinical course
Nodular	Adult	0.5–5+	Distal lower extremity	Often numerous	Rare	Rare	Relatively indolent
Florid-infiltrating	Adult	1–5+	Distal extremities most common	Few	Common	Common	Relatively aggressive
Lymphadenopathic	Children	Nodes massively enlarged	All nodal groups	Numerous	No	No	Rapid fatality

HISTOPATHOLOGIC VARIANTS

Three histopathologic variants of Kaposi's sarcoma are recognized. Seen to varying degrees in all populations affected, these include a spindle cell variant, a mixed cell type, and an anaplastic form (Table 2) (3,4,6,7).

Spindle cell Kaposi's sarcoma presents a bland uniform population of elongated cells. Mitoses are rare, and clinical behavior is often indolent.

Mixed cell types of Kaposi's sarcoma are recognized by a combination of spindle cells and a proliferation of vascular structures, often with large malignant-appearing endothelial cells, and by an extravasation of erythrocytes. Mixed cell tumors are common in all clinical settings, particularly in patients with AIDS. Because of extravasation of erythrocytes into the tumor and beyond the tumor into adjacent normal skin, ecchymosis is often observed during physical examination. The clinical course of mixed cell Kaposi's sarcoma is frequently more aggressive than the spindle cell variant.

Anaplastic tumors of Kaposi's sarcoma are often seen in the florid and infiltrating variants of African Kaposi's sarcoma. Anaplastic tumors are histologically characterized by an extremely undifferentiated uniform cell population with frequent mitoses.

Table 2 Histologic Variants of Kaposi's Sarcoma

Type	Clinical variant	Brief description
Mixed cell	Nodular, lymphadenopathic	Combined populations of spindle-shaped cells and vascular proliferations lined by large endothelial cells
Spindle cell	Nodular	Bland, uniform population of elongated cells; mitoses rare
Anaplastic	Florid-infiltrating	Disordered growth of large undifferentiated cells

CLINICAL FEATURES IN NON-AIDS POPULATIONS

Classic Kaposi's sarcoma seen in the elderly population is initially recognized by cutaneous nodules primarily affecting the skin of the distal lower extremities (Table 3) (4). These nodule tumors may be of the mixed or spindle cell histopathologic variants. The median age of onset is greater than 70 years, and men are affected 14 times as frequently as women. The clinical course of classic Kaposi's sarcoma is usually indolent. The median duration of survival is 8–13 years, and the tumor remains confined to the skin until later in the course of disease when visceral spread may occur. Because of the advanced age of affected patients and the indolent clinical course, classic Kaposi's sarcoma is usually not the direct cause of death and often does not require specific therapy. There is no specific immune deficiency associated with classic Kaposi's sarcoma apart from the expected immune attrition of aging. Patients with classic Kaposi's sarcoma are not prone to opportunistic infections and are not infected with the human immunodeficiency virus (HIV) (9).

Table 3 Kaposi's Sarcoma in Non-AIDS Populations

Group	Age	Sex	Course	Immune deficits
Classic	70+	M-F $\geq$ 15:1	Indolent	No
African (prior to 1975)	Children to young adults	M-F $\simeq$ 1.0	Variable	No
Exogenously immune deficient	Adults	M-F $\simeq$ 1	Aggressive (response to decrease in immune deficiency)	Yes: iatrogenic

African Kaposi's sarcoma was recognized and reported well before the appearance of HIV. African Kaposi's sarcoma has been common in the parts of Africa now affected by AIDS, and further confusion is generated by the recognition of aggressive Kaposi's sarcoma in these same parts of Africa, which now appear to be associated with infection of HIV.

African Kaposi's sarcoma before the AIDS epidemic took many clinical and histopathologic forms (3,10,11). Nodular lesions were common, but florid and infiltrating lesions were also observed and children were particularly affected by the lymphadenopathic clinical variant. Spindle cell and mixed cell tumors were seen in the nodular forms, and the florid and infiltrating Kaposi's tumors were frequently anaplastic.

The natural history of these variants of African Kaposi's sarcoma is rather distinct (11–13). Nodular forms, usually seen in adults, have a relatively indolent course compared with florid tumors, which often progress rapidly, causing local tissue destruction and when compared with lymphadenopathic Kaposi's in the young, which has a high and rapid mortality rate and a less substantial response to therapeutic intervention.

African Kaposi's sarcoma, prior to the mid-1970s, was not associated with underlying immune deficiency or with HIV infection (12–15). The only reported immunodeficiency occurred in patients with far advanced disease and is probably comparable to that seen in other patients with advanced cancers. Opportunistic infections were not reported to be increased in African Kaposi's sarcoma, and response to therapy was often much more gratifying than in current cases in patients with AIDS.

KAPOSI'S SARCOMA IN THE IATROGENICALLY IMMUNOSUPPRESSED

With the advent of the more widespread use of powerful immunosuppressing agents in organ transplantation and in the treatment of autoimmune disorders came the recognition that this therapy was associated with an increased risk of cancers. Kaposi's sarcoma is one of the cancers most often seen in immunosuppressed individuals and may develop rather quickly after renal transplantation (16–21).

Nodular forms predominate in the immunosuppressed Kaposi's sarcoma patient, but early visceral involvement is frequent. The most common of the histopathologic variants, the mixed cell type, is most frequently seen in renal transplant patients. The median age of Kaposi's sarcoma patients in this setting reflects that of organ transplantation, being much younger than classic Kaposi's sarcoma. Also in contrast to classic Kaposi's sarcoma, any site of the body may be affected by Kaposi's sarcoma in the organ transplant recipient, and the clinical course is characterized by rapid tumor progression. Of interest and of importance to our approach to Kaposi's sarcoma in patients with AIDS, the tumor has been reported to regress when iatrogenic immunosuppression can be withdrawn, allowing restoration of normal host defenses (21–23).

AIDS-RELATED KAPOSI'S SARCOMA

Beginning in 1980 and reported in mid-1981, Kaposi's sarcoma began to be diagnosed in young male homosexuals in the United States (24–26). The previous rarity of the tumor in young men was one of the early indications of appearance of the AIDS epidemic. Kaposi's sarcoma has remained the most common AIDS-related neoplasm, and the ease of diagnosis has facilitated our understanding of the spread of the AIDS epidemic, especially in the homosexual community in the United States. It was also the recognition of Kaposi's sarcoma in Haitians that led to wider appreciation of the international occurrence of the AIDS epidemic (11,13,27–29).

Kaposi's sarcoma represents many unique features in the setting of AIDS (Table 4). AIDS patients may have each of the clinical variants of Kaposi's sarcoma seen in other populations, but nodular lesions predominate. In contrast, however, to the nodular tumor in classic Kaposi's sarcoma, patients with AIDS often have lymphatic

Table 4 Clinical Features of Kaposi's Sarcoma in AIDS

Most common in *homosexual* AIDS patients
Nodular, mixed cell tumors
Widely disseminated, all body regions (especially face, oral cavity)
Visceral spread common even early in disease course
Severe underlying immune deficiency with death from opportunistic infections
Response to therapy: incomplete and brief

involvement. Visceral involvement, particularly of the gastrointestinal tract, is also not uncommon even early in the course of the disease. Although most patients with AIDS-related Kaposi's sarcoma do have cutaneous lesions, other patients have disease confined to the lymph nodes or to visceral structures. The most common histopathologic variant in patients with AIDS is the mixed cell type. Extravasation of erythrocytes into normal skin is often striking and may herald the appearance of typical cutaneous nodules. Patients with AIDS-related Kaposi's sarcoma are young, with a median age of 35 years. Kaposi's sarcoma in AIDS is relatively confined to homosexual men for reasons that are not yet completely understood but that may involve differential exposure to sexually transmitted viruses, such as cytomegalovirus, or the use of recreational drugs, such as amyl nitrites (30–33).

Any site of the body may be affected by AIDS-related Kaposi's sarcoma, and the head and neck are frequently involved, in distinct contrast to most other forms of this tumor (34,35) [Figures 3 and 4 (see Plates I and II, facing pp. 178–179)]. Also in contrast to classic Kaposi's sarcoma, the tumor in AIDS is rarely confined to a single anatomic region. Kaposi's sarcoma appears to be multicentric; tumors in the same stage of development appear in widely separated regions of the body. Tumors are pigmented and usually painless and nonpruritic and are rarely exophytic. Kaposi's sarcoma lesions in AIDS patients may be strikingly symmetrical and are often linear, following cutaneous lymphatic drainage [Figure 5 (see Plate II, facing p. 179)]. For reasons not yet clearly understood, the soles of the feet are commonly affected, but the palms are rarely involved. Some other common sites of disease include the tip of the nose, the region behind the ear, the conjunctiva, the oral mucosa, and the penis.

The course of AIDS-related Kaposi's sarcoma is extremely variable. For example, patients with minimal disease and no symptoms suggestive of other underlying infectious disease have an excellent 5-year survival rate. Usually, however, patients with Kaposi's sarcoma in the setting of HIV infection have a rapid progression of their cancer with visceral involvement similar to that seen in patients who are iatrogenically immunosuppressed. Even given this rapid progression, however, Kaposi's sarcoma is uncommonly the primary cause of death in AIDS when compared with the frequency of death following specific opportunistic infections.

A variety of clinical syndromes of Kaposi's sarcoma are seen in patients with AIDS that deserve further elaboration. These include the oral manifestations of this tumor, its appearance in the lymph nodes, visceral Kaposi's sarcoma, and tumor-associated lymphedema.

ORAL KAPOSI'S SARCOMA

As many as one-third of patients with AIDS-related Kaposi's sarcoma have oral involvement at the time of diagnosis (36,37) [Figures 6A,B (See Plate II, facing p. 179)]. Kaposi's sarcoma lesions in the oral cavity typically affect the mucosa of the hard and soft palate and, less commonly, the posterior pharyngeal wall or the tonsillar pillars. Although the gingiva is not uncommonly affected, the buccal mucosa, tongue, and floor of the mouth are rarely involved.

Similar to other cutaneous sites, oral Kaposi's sarcoma appears as a red to blue discoloration ranging from several millimeters to one or more centimeters in diameter. Nodularity is a less striking feature of oral Kaposi's sarcoma, although the tumor later in the course of disease may become bulky and in advanced cases necrosis

PLATE I
(Chapter 7)

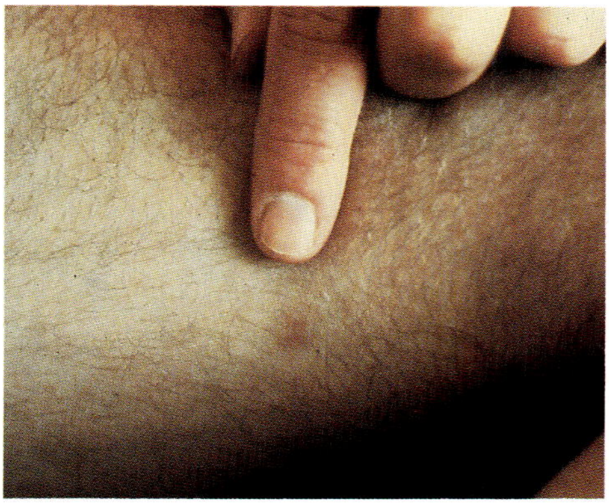

Figure 1A Early lesion of Kaposi's sarcoma—nodular variant in AIDS.

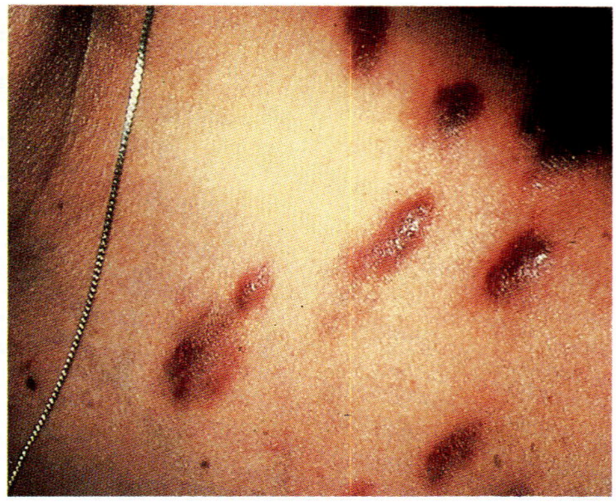

Figure 1B Nodular Kaposi's sarcoma in subclavicular distribution.

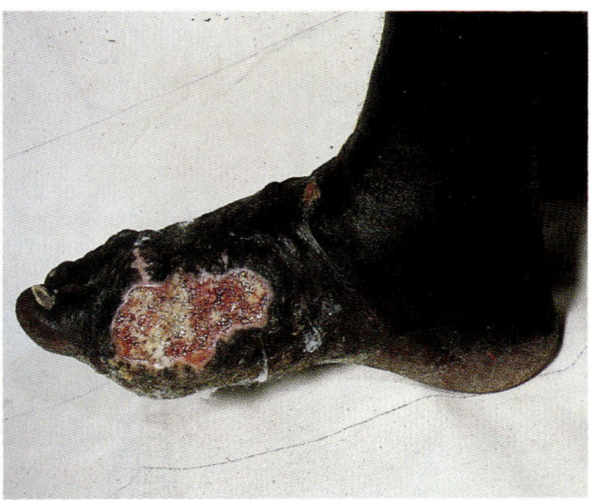

Figure 2 Infiltrating or florid Kaposi's sarcoma of lower extremity in African (non-AIDS) patient. (Courtesy of Dr. John L. Ziegler.)

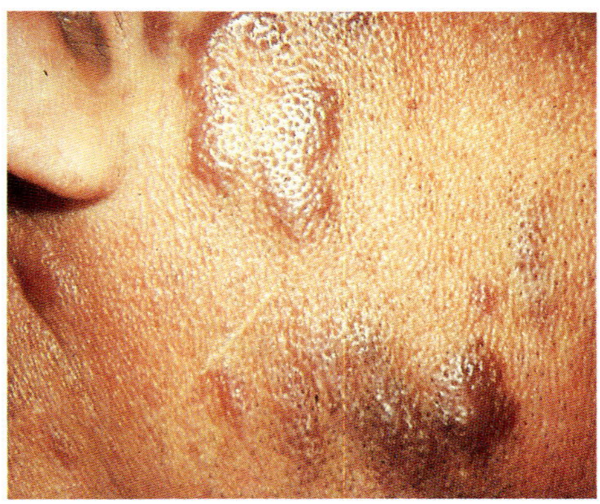

Figure 3 Large nodular Kaposi's sarcoma lesion on face of patient with AIDS.

PLATE II
(*Chapter 7*)

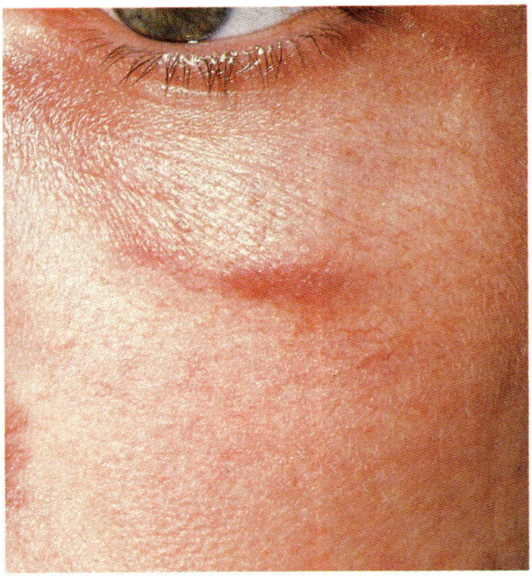

Figure 4 Facial nodular lesion of AIDS-related Kaposi's sarcoma. Facial involvement is often accompanied by lymphedema later in the disease course.

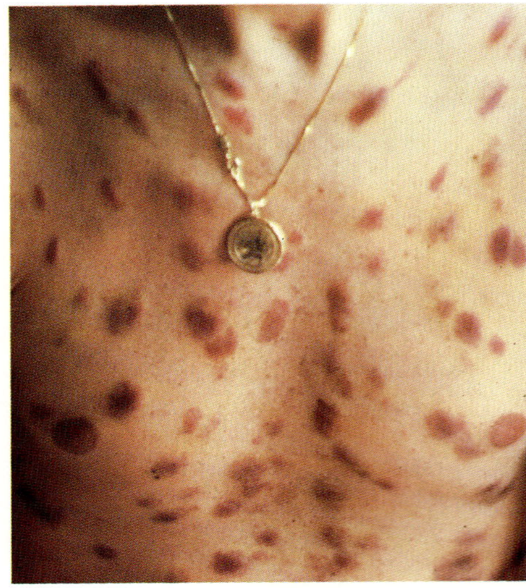

Figure 5 Truncal Kaposi's sarcoma lesions in AIDS patient illustrating symmetry and linearity common in this distribution.

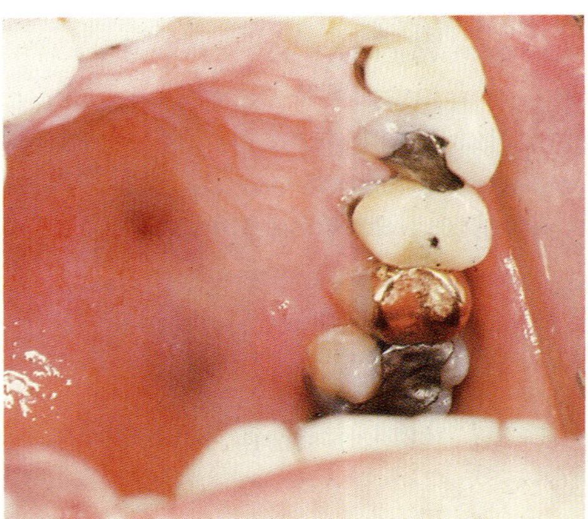

Figure 6A Kaposi's sarcoma involving the hard palate—the most common site of oral involvement.

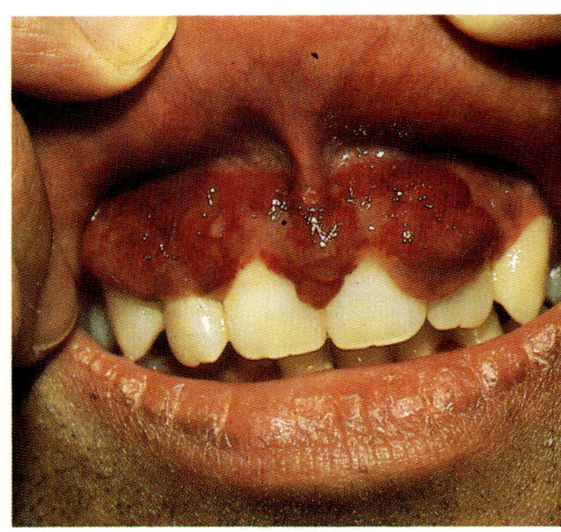

Figure 6B Extensive gingival Kaposi's sarcoma in AIDS.

may occur. Oral lesions are generally asymptomatic except large tumors, which may obstruct swallowing or cause pain.

LYMPHATIC INVOLVEMENT

Early in the recognition of patients with AIDS-related Kaposi's sarcoma, it was appreciated that lymph nodes could be enlarged and when biopsied often contained foci of Kaposi's sarcoma (35, 38–40). These foci range from small deposits that require careful sectioning to detect to entire replacement of nodes in any body site. Lymph node biopsy was typically performed in Kaposi's sarcoma patients but is now less often required given better recognition of cutaneous lesions and because lymphatic involvement is not associated with a substantially worse prognosis.

VISCERAL INVOLVEMENT

Visceral involvement, like lymphatic, is common in AIDS patients with Kaposi's sarcoma. The gastrointestinal tract, when explored carefully, may be found to be affected in as many as 50% of patients even early in the course of disease (40–42). Any site of the gastrointestinal tract from the oral mucosa to the rectum may be affected, but the most common site is the small bowel, especially the duodenum.

Despite the typical appearance on endoscopy of vascular, nodular lesions, biopsies are diagnostic in only 23% of cases because the tumors are submucosal (42). This location may also help explain the infrequency of clinical bleeding associated with gastrointestinal tract involvement. Obstruction is also rare, but extensive gastrointestinal tract involvement may be associated with enteropathy and with the diarrhea so often problematic in AIDS patients.

Pulmonary spread is less commonly recognized in AIDS patients than is gastrointestinal. The lung is typically involved late in the course of the disease. Its diagnosis may be difficult because of similarities radiologically and clinically with pulmonary opportunistic infections. Pulmonary Kaposi's sarcoma, however, is generally not a cause of diffuse pulmonary uptake on gallium scanning, and pleural effusions common in pulmonary Kaposi's sarcoma are rare in other pulmonary manifestations of AIDS. Pulmonary Kaposi's sarcoma is associated with a rapid mortality from respiratory insufficiency with a median survival in some series as short as 2 months (43–46).

Pulmonary Kaposi's sarcoma is diagnosed by excluding common pulmonary opportunistic infections and by documenting the typical appearance of endobronchial Kaposi's sarcoma lesions, which appear as small vascular nodules lining the tracheobronchial tree. Because of fear of hemorrhage, biopsy is usually not performed.

ASSOCIATED LYMPHEDEMA

Because Kaposi's sarcoma appears to arise from lymphatic endothelium, lymphedema should not be an unexpected sequella. Lymphedema is often striking and is most commonly seen in the face, causing disfiguration. Facial lymphedema may be so striking as to obstruct vision and hearing. Lymphedema both in the face and in the lower extremities, where it is also extremely common, may occur out of proportion to the extent of cutaneous tumors. This reflects an obliteration of small cutaneous lymphatics and may help explain the lack of success of regional therapies, such as radiation treatment.

STAGING AIDS-RELATED KAPOSI'S SARCOMA

The reasons for developing an accurate staging system for AIDS related Kaposi's sarcoma are numerous. They include an improvement in our ability to discuss prognosis with individual patients. Staging systems can also improve the selection of appropriate candidates for experimental trials and can greatly improve our ability to compare the results of clinical trials conducted in different centers.

Many difficulties have surrounded the development of staging systems of AIDS-related Kaposi's sarcoma. These include the relative newness of this disease and the many unique features of Kaposi's sarcoma in AIDS patients compared with other populations. Another difficulty is the extreme variability in the clinical course, which may reflect variations in the underlying level of immune dysfunction instead of usual estimates of tumor burden. Finally, the lack of staging systems reflects an insufficient attention given to this important problem compared with the amount of effort expended on developing and testing experimental agents.

Despite the difficulties involved, some information has accrued regarding the staging of AIDS-related Kaposi's sarcoma. Probably the most widely accepted system has been proposed by investigators at New York University (Table 5) (47). They have used a four-stage system with staging based on the clinical ap-

Table 5 Clinical Staging of Kaposi's Sarcoma

Tumor extent
Stage I: cutaneous, locally indolent
Stage II: cutaneous, locally aggressive, with or without regional lymph nodes
Stage III: generalized[a] mucocutaneous and/or lymph node involvement
Stage IV: visceral
Symptomatic status
A: asymptomatic
B: systemic signs: weight loss (10%); fever (>100°F) orally, unrelated to an identifiable source of infection, lasting > 2 weeks

[a]Generalized means more than upper or lower extremities alone: includes minimal gastrointestinal disease defined as fewer than five lesions, <2 cm in *combined diameters*.

pearance of the tumor and tumor involvement of internal organs. In this system, stage I is defined as cutaneous, locally indolent, or classic variant Kaposi's sarcoma; stage II is cutaneous and locally aggressive with or without regional lymph nodes, as is typical in African, locally aggressive tumors; stage III is generalized cutaneous or lymph node involvement; and stage IV is visceral Kaposi's sarcoma. In addition to the four staging classes, subtypes A and B are defined by the absence or presence, respectively, of systemic symptoms, including unexplained weight loss, persistent fevers, or night sweats.

The NYU staging system has been widely used, although there are certain problems with this system. For example, only two of the four stages relate directly to Kaposi's sarcoma as seen in patients with AIDS, namely, stages III and IV. Also, when survival of the various stages is examined, it is apparent that there is no survival difference between stages III and IV, but there is a substantial difference between those patients with or without systemic signs. Therefore, in practical terms, this is only a two-stage system and is not extremely helpful for detailed comparison of clinical trial results.

Another attempt to define prognostic variables in Kaposi's sarcoma was developed in San Francisco (48,49). Here, clinical and routine laboratory findings were analyzed for effect on survival. Although still incompletely developed, this work suggests that in addition to systemic signs, routine laboratory abnormalities are also prognostically significant. For example, the survival in patients with erythrocyte sedimentation rates (ESR) greater than 40 mm/hour was significantly reduced compared with that in patients with lower ESR. Also patients with cytopenias, particularly granulocytopenia, have shortened survival. Again, this staging system is of limited practical application but does suggest areas for additional refinement in the clinical staging of Kaposi's sarcoma.

The final area of work in the staging of Kaposi's sarcoma has focused on immunologic variables. Work in both Los Angeles (50) and New York (51) has correlated survival with degree of immune deficiency. For example, the survival of patients with absolute number of circulating T-helper cells of less than 100 cells/mm^2 is substantially worse than patients with 100–400 cells/mm^2. The survival of patients with more than 400 cells/mm^2 is in turn significantly longer than the other two groups. Functional immunologic assays have also been shown to be of importance, with decreased mitogen responsiveness also correlating with a poorer survival.

Considering the importance of developing an accurate staging and prognostic classification system for AIDS-related Kaposi's sarcoma, the deficiencies in the studies just discussed are grounds for concern. Clearly, a major effort must be undertaken to develop and validate—using both retrospective and prospective information—an accurate staging system for this important disease. In the interim, it seems prudent to combine elements of the staging research that has been conducted.

Although it is difficult to quantitate precisely the tumor burden, it does seem important to include in a staging system some estimate of this variable. This can take the form of arbitrary grouping of patients by the number of cutaneous lesions or by the extent of the body area involved with this disease. Routine endoscopic evaluation is not performed in most centers, but it seems appropriate to classify patients with known visceral involvement in a worse prognostic group. Of more importance are the presence or absence of lymphoma-like B symptoms, including night sweats, fevers, and weight loss. As these are the most important variables affecting survival that have been identified to date, these signs or their absence must be recorded in any clinical trial report. For laboratory studies, the absolute number of T-helper cells seems to be the most important variable and also should be included in staging systems.

The composite of these recommendations would suggest that a staging system to be validated should separate patients as to tumor burden (minimal or advanced), systemic signs (absent or present), and absolute number of T-helper cells (<100, $<100–400$, >400). It is hoped that validation of such a system will proceed rapidly.

REFERENCES

1. Kaposi M. Idiopathisiches multiples pigmensarkom der haut. Arch Dermatol Syph (Berlin) 1872; 4:265.
2. Odajnyk C, Muggia F. Treatment of Kaposi's sarcoma: overview and analysis by clinical setting. J Clin Oncol 1985; 3:1277–85.
3. Taylor J, Templeton A, Vogel C, et al. Kaposi's sarcoma in Uganda: a clinico-pathological study. Int J Cancer 1971; 8:122–35.
4. Safai B, Good R. Kaposi's sarcoma: a review and recent developments. CA 1981; 31:2–12.
5. Olweny C, Kaddumukasa A, Atine I, et al. Childhood Kaposi's sarcoma: clinical features and therapy. Cancer 1976; 33:555–60.
6. Su I-J, Kuo T-T, Wu S-Y, et al. Lymphadenopathic type of Kaposi's sarcoma presenting with generalized petechial hemorrhages—a case report from Taiwan. Cancer 1984; 54:948–50.
7. McNutt NS, Fletcher V, Conant M. Early lesions of Kaposi's sarcoma in homosexual men. An ultrastructural comparison with other vascular proliferations in skin. Am J Pathol 1983; 111:62–77.
8. Dorfman R. Kaposi's sarcoma revisited. Hum Pathol 1984; 15:1013–17.
9. Marinig C, Fiorini G, Boneschi V, et al. Immunologic and immunogenetic features of primary Kaposi's sarcoma. Cancer 1985; 55:1899–1901.
10. Weber J. Is acquired immune deficiency syndrome an epidemic form of African Kaposi's sarcoma? Discussion paper. J R Soc Med 1984; 77:July.
11. Bayley A, Downing R, Cheingsong-Popov R, et al. HTLV-III serology distinguishes atypical and endemic Kaposi's sarcoma in Africa. Lancet February 16 1985; 359–61.
12. Bayley AC. Aggressive Kaposi's sarcoma in Zambia, 1983. Lancet June 16, 1984; 1318–22.
13. Biggar R. The acquired immune deficiency syndrome problem in Africa. Lancet January 11, 1986; 79–82.
14. Keystens L, Melbye M, Biggar R, et al. Endemic African Kaposi's sarcoma is not associated with immunodeficiency. Int J Cancer 1985; 36:49–54.
15. Master S, Taylor J, Kyalwazi S, et al. Immunological studies in Kaposi's sarcoma in Uganda. Br Med J 1970; 1–8.
16. Meyers A, Rice G, Kay S, et al. Kaposi's sarcoma in an immunosuppressed renal allograft recipient. S Afr Med J July 1976; 1299–1300.

17. Hoshaw R, Schwartz R. Kaposi's sarcoma after immunosuppressive therapy with prednisone. Arch Dermatol 1980; 116:1280.
18. Krueger T, Tallent M, Richie R, et al. Neoplasia in immunosuppressed renal transplant patients: a 20 year experience. South Med J 1985; 78:501–6.
19. Siegel J, Janis R, Alper J, et al. Disseminated visceral Kaposi's sarcoma: appearance after human renal homograft operation. JAMA 1969; 207:1493–6.
20. Klepp O, Dahl O, Trygve-Stenwig J. Association of Kaposi's sarcoma and prior immunosuppressive therapy. Cancer 1978; 42:2626.
21. Zisbrod Z, Haimov M, Schanzer H, et al. Kaposi's sarcoma after kidney transplantation. Report of complete remission of cutaneous and visceral involvement. Transplantation 1980; 30:383–4.
22. Stribling J, Weitzner S, Smith G. Kaposi's sarcoma in renal allograft recipients. Cancer 1978; 42:442–6.
23. Little P, Farthing C, Khader A, et al. Kaposi's sarcoma in a patient after renal transplantation. Postgrad Med J 1983; 59:325–6.
24. Moss A, Bacchetti P, Osmond D, et al. Incidence of the acquired immune deficiency syndrome in San Francisco. 1980–83. J Infect Dis 1985; 152:152–61.
25. Friedman-Kien A, Laubenstein L, Rubeinstein P, et al. Disseminated Kaposi's sarcoma in homosexual men. Ann Intern Med 1982; 96:693–700.
26. Haverkos H, Drotman D, Morgan M. Prevalence of Kaposi's sarcoma among patients with AIDS (letter). N Engl J Med 1985; 312:1518.
27. Pape J, Liautaud B, Thomas F, et al. The acquired immunodeficiency syndrome in Haiti. Ann Intern Med 1985; 103:674–8.
28. Pitchenik A, Fischl M, Dickinson G, et al. Opportunistic infections and Kaposi's sarcoma among Haitians: evidence of a new acquired immunodeficiency state. Ann Intern Med 1983; 98:277–84.
29. Pape J, Liautaud B, Thomas F, et al. Characteristics of the acquired immunodeficiency syndrome (AIDS) in Haiti. N Engl J Med 1983; 309:945–50.
30. Cohn D, Judson F. Absence of Kaposi's sarcoma in hemophiliacs with the acquired immune deficiency syndrome (letter). Ann Intern Med 1984; 101:401.
31. Guinan M, Thomas P, Pinsky P, et al. Heterosexual and homosexual patients with acquired immune deficiency syndrome. Ann Intern Med 1984; 100:213–8.

32. Newell G, Adams S, Mansell P, et al. Toxicity, immunosuppressive effects and carcinogenic potential of volatile nitrites: possible relationship to Kaposi's sarcoma. Pharmacotherapy 1984; 4:284–91.
33. Marmor M, Friedman-Kien A, Laubenstein L, et al. Risk factors for Kaposi's sarcoma in homosexual men. Lancet 1982; 1:1083–86.
34. Rosenberg R, Schneider K, Cohen N. Head and neck presentations of acquired immune deficiency syndrome. Otolaryngol Head Neck Surg 1985; 93:700.
35. Safai B, Sarngadharan M, Koziner B, et al. Spectrum of Kaposi's sarcoma in the epidemic of acquired immune deficiency syndrome. Cancer 1985; 45:4646–8.
36. Lozada F, Silverman S, Migliorati C, et al. Oral manifestations of tumor and opportunistic infections in the acquired immune deficiency syndrome: findings in 53 homosexual men with Kaposi's sarcoma. Oral Surg 1983; 56:491–94.
37. Green T, Beckstead J, Lozada-Nur F, et al. Histopathologic spectrum of oral Kaposi's sarcoma. Oral Surg 1984; 58:306–14.
38. Boyko W, Sharp F, Jeffries E, et al. Small foci of Kaposi's sarcoma in lymph nodes may be missed without serial sections (letter). Lancet 1984; 1:158.
39. Abrams DI. AIDS-related lymphadenopathy: the role of biopsy. J Clin Oncol 1986; 4:126–7.
40. Reichert CM, O'Leary TJ, Levens DL, et al. Autopsy pathology in the acquired immune deficiency syndrome. Am J Pathol 1983; 112:357.
41. Rose H, Balthazar E, Megibow A, et al. Alimentary tract involvement in Kaposi's sarcoma: radiographic and endoscopic findings in 25 homosexual men. Am J Radiol 1982; 139:661–6.
42. Friedman S, Wright T, Altman D. Gastrointestinal Kaposi's sarcoma in patients with acquired immunodeficiency syndrome. Endoscopic and autopsy findings. Gastroenterology 1985; 89:102–8.
43. Nash G, Fligiel S. Kaposi's sarcoma presenting as pulmonary disease in the acquired immune deficiency syndrome: diagnosis by lung biopsy. Hum Pathol 1984; 15:999.
44. Meduri G, Stover D, Lee M, et al. Pulmonary Kaposi's sarcoma in the acquired immune deficiency syndrome. Am J Med 1986; 81:11–8.
45. Rucker L, Meador J. Kaposi's sarcoma presenting as homogeneous pulmonary infiltrates in a patient with acquired immunodeficiency syndrome. West J Med 1985; 142:831–3.
46. Ognibene F, Steis R, Macher A, et al. Kaposi's sarcoma causing

pulmonary infiltrates and respiratory failure in acquired immune deficiency syndrome. Ann Intern Med 1985; 102:471–5.
47. Krigel R, Laubenstein L, Muggia F. Kaposi's sarcoma: a new staging classification. Cancer Treat Rep 1983; 67:531–4.
48. Volberding P, Kaslow K, Bilk M, et al. Prognostic factors in staging Kaposi's sarcoma in the acquired immune deficiency syndrome (abstract). Am Soc Clin Oncol 1984; 3:51.
49. Cutler K, Feigal D, Hearst N, et al. Prognostic indicators at presentation of Kaposi's sarcoma (abstract). Submitted (1987) to III International Conference on AIDS, Washington, D.C.
50. Taylor J, Afrasiabi R, Fahey J, et al. Prognostically significant classification of immune changes in acquired immune deficiency syndrome with Kaposi's sarcoma. Blood 1986; 67:666–71.
51. Vadhan-Raj S, Wong G, Gnecco C, et al. Immunological variables as predictors of prognosis in patients with Kaposi's sarcoma and acquired immune deficiency syndrome. Cancer Res 1976; 46:417–25.

8

Radiologic Features

Susan D. Wall
Veterans Administration Medical Center
and University of California
San Francisco, California

Traditionally, the radiography of Kaposi's sarcoma was limited primarily to angiography of soft tissue nodules, plain films of the skeleton, and occasionally lymphangiography (1–4). None of these procedures plays a current role in the diagnostic evaluation of Kaposi's sarcoma, since the onset of the acquired immunodeficiency syndrome (AIDS) epidemic. Angiography and lymphangiography are not useful diagnostically and cystic bony lesions detected by plain films of the skeleton are not encountered in AIDS-associated Kaposi's sarcoma. With classic or even the more aggressive African Kaposi's sarcoma, lytic lesions in the skeleton were present only in the setting of advanced disease (2). This chapter discusses the utility of various current imaging techniques in the diagnosis of AIDS-associated Kaposi's sarcoma in the abdomen, chest, and head. The major radiographic features are summarized in Table 1.

Table 1 Radiographic Signs That Suggest Kaposi's Sarcoma

Gastrointestinal tract
Nodules (± central umbilication)
Coalescent masses
Asymmetric thickening
Multifocal lesions
Abdominal computed tomography
Lymphadenopathy > 1.0–1.5 cm
Lymphadenopathy with central low density
Decreased density of enlarged muscle
Increased density of fat (diffuse or focal)
Asymmetric thickening of gastrointestinal tract
Low-density lesions in solid organ
Lung
Parenchymal nodules
Pleural effusion
Intracerebral (insufficient data)

GASTROINTESTINAL RADIOGRAPHY

Barium Radiography

Barium contrast radiographs are helpful in the diagnostic evaluation of patients with suspected gastrointestinal Kaposi's sarcoma and can be directive when diagnosis requires visual inspection by endoscopy or colonoscopy. Gastrointestinal Kaposi's sarcoma, which may antedate skin or lymph node involvement in patients with AIDS, has been noted in all parts of the gastrointestinal tract. Its endoscopic appearance of red-purple or violaceous lesions is so characteristic as to no longer require biopsy for diagnosis (5). Moreover, biopsy of the early lesions often is falsely negative (6) because the forceps of the flexible fiberoptic endoscope usually do not reach the submucosa where the tumor originates.

Early Kaposi's sarcoma lesions seen on endoscopy are macular and thus are not demonstrated on barium radiography of the intestinal mucosa. As the lesions progress, they become nodular and then are well demonstrated in the stomach (Figure 1), duodenum, and colon (Figure 2) on double-contrast barium examination (7–10). Occasionally, central umbilication may be seen, but the presence of "target" or "bull's-eye" lesions is not essential for the radiographic diagnosis of Kaposi's sarcoma. With further progression of disease, the lesions enlarge and may coalesce (Figures 3 and 4), sometimes causing gastric outlet or duodenal obstruction (Figure 5). Large rectosigmoid masses are not uncommon in advanced disease (Figure 6).

Small bowel involvement generally is manifested by diffuse fold thickening, which may be regular or irregular, focal or diffuse (Figure 7). Nodularity may be present, and uncommonly, tumor nodules may cause small bowel intussusception (Figure 8) or acute appendicitis. The small bowel findings on barium radiography are not specific for Kaposi's sarcoma, and the differential diagnosis includes inflammatory bowel disease and other tumors (see below). Opportunistic infections, such as with monilial enteritis (11) and cytomegalovirus gastroenteritis (12), cause similar findings of fold thickening. Cryptosporidiosis also can cause fold thickening

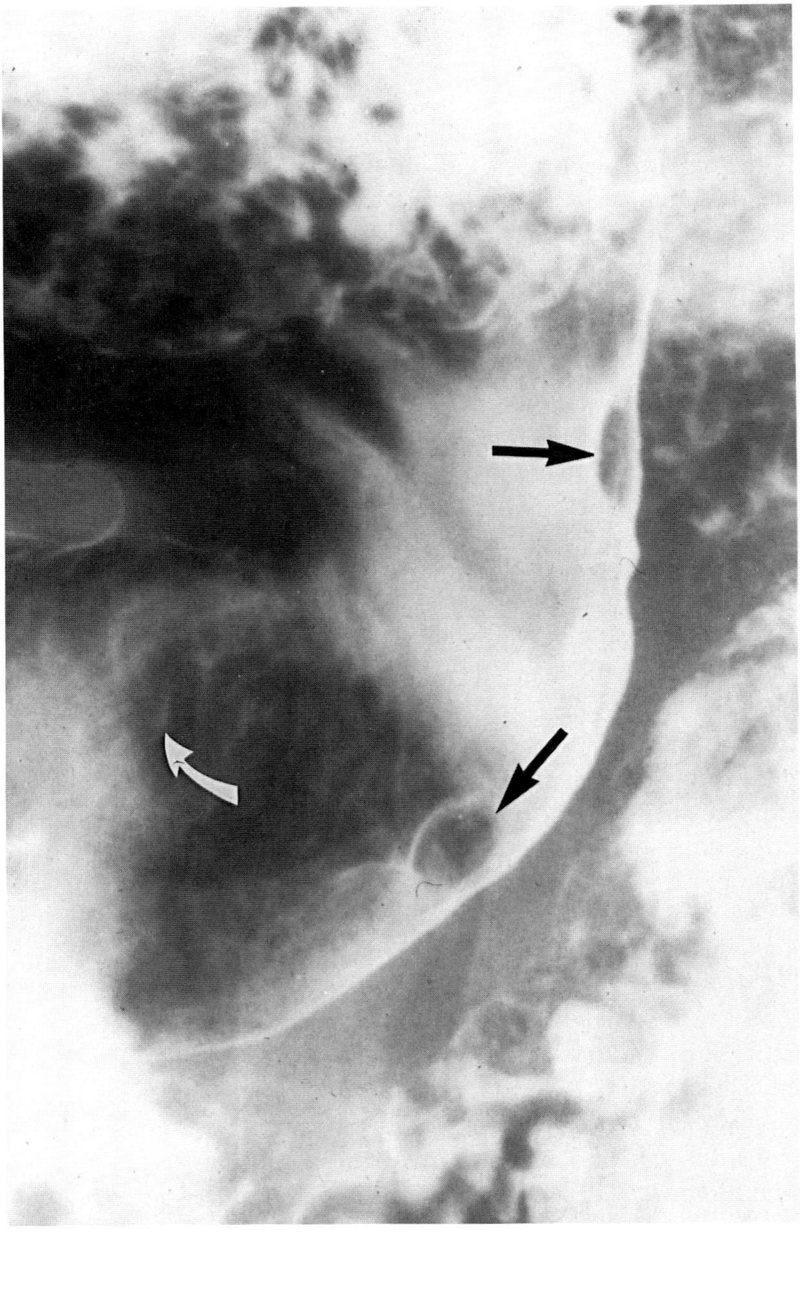

Figure 1 Early gastrointestinal Kaposi's sarcoma. Double-contrast barium examination demonstrates nodular lesions (black arrows) of early Kaposi's sarcoma in the gastric antrum of this 37-year-old homosexual man with AIDS. Central umbilication (curved white arrow) is seen, but such "target" or "bull's-eye" lesions are only occasionally present. (Reproduced from References 9 and 14 with permission.)

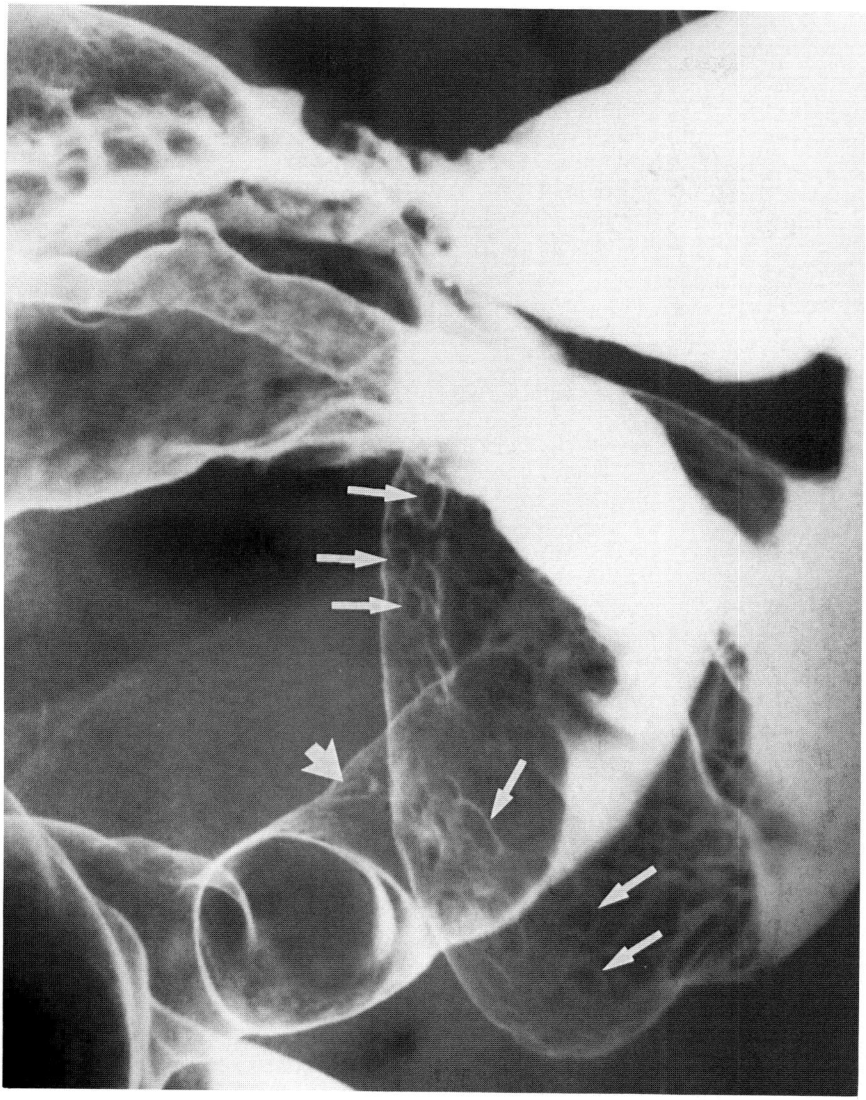

Figure 2 Early colonic Kaposi's sarcoma. Double-contrast barium enema demonstrates early nodular lesions (arrows) of Kaposi's sarcoma. Central umbilication is noted in one lesion only (arrowhead); it is not commonly demonstrated radiographically. (Reproduced from Reference 7 with permission.)

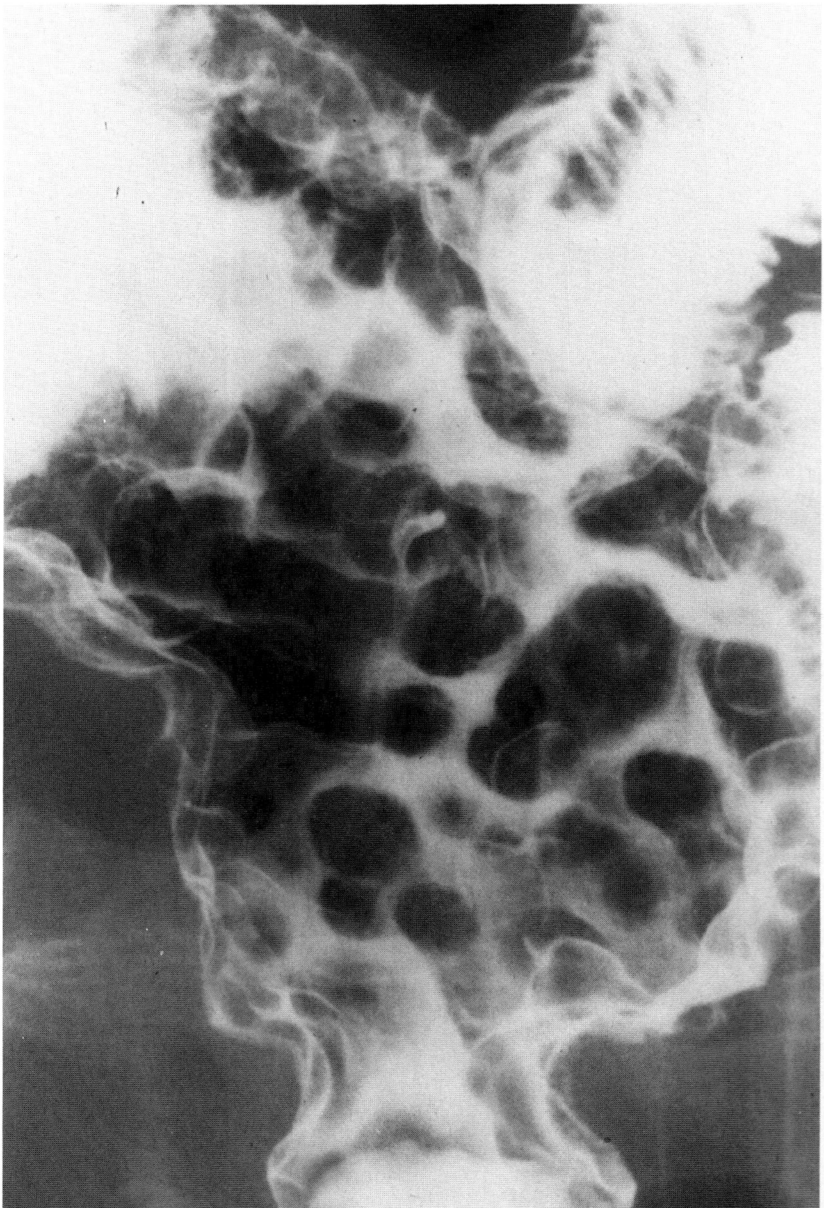

Figure 3 Advanced gastrointestinal Kaposi's sarcoma. The same patient as in Figure 1, reimaged 6 months later. Multiple nodular masses of advanced Kaposi's sarcoma are present throughout the entire stomach. (Reproduced from reference 14 with permission.)

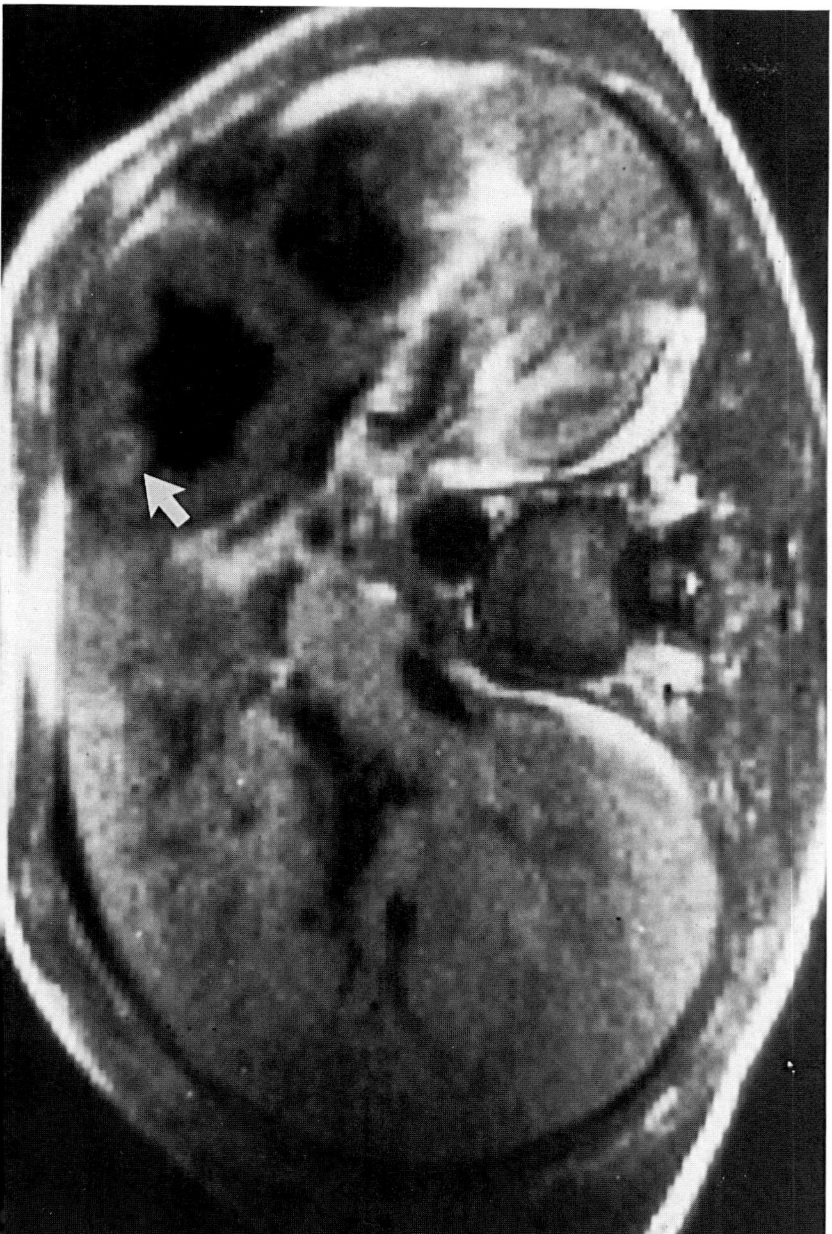

Figure 4 Kaposi's sarcoma of the stomach. Transverse magnetic resonance image of the stomach demonstrates diffuse nodular thickening due to Kaposi's sarcoma in a homosexual man with AIDS. The thickened gastric wall is normal in signal intensity, except for several focal areas of increased signal intensity (arrow), possibly due to the vascularity of this tumor.

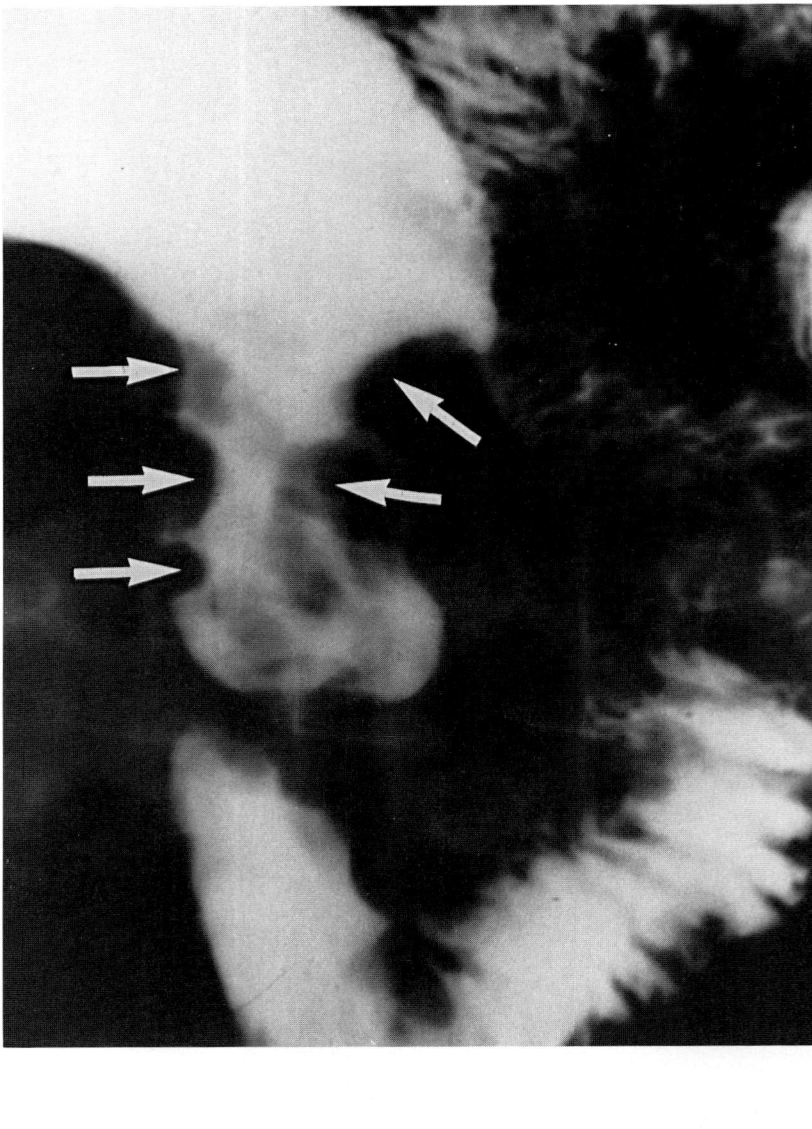

Figure 5 Advanced gastric Kaposi's sarcoma. Single-contrast barium examination demonstrates bulky tumor masses (arrows) of Kaposi's sarcoma causing incomplete gastric outlet obstruction; radiation therapy was palliative.

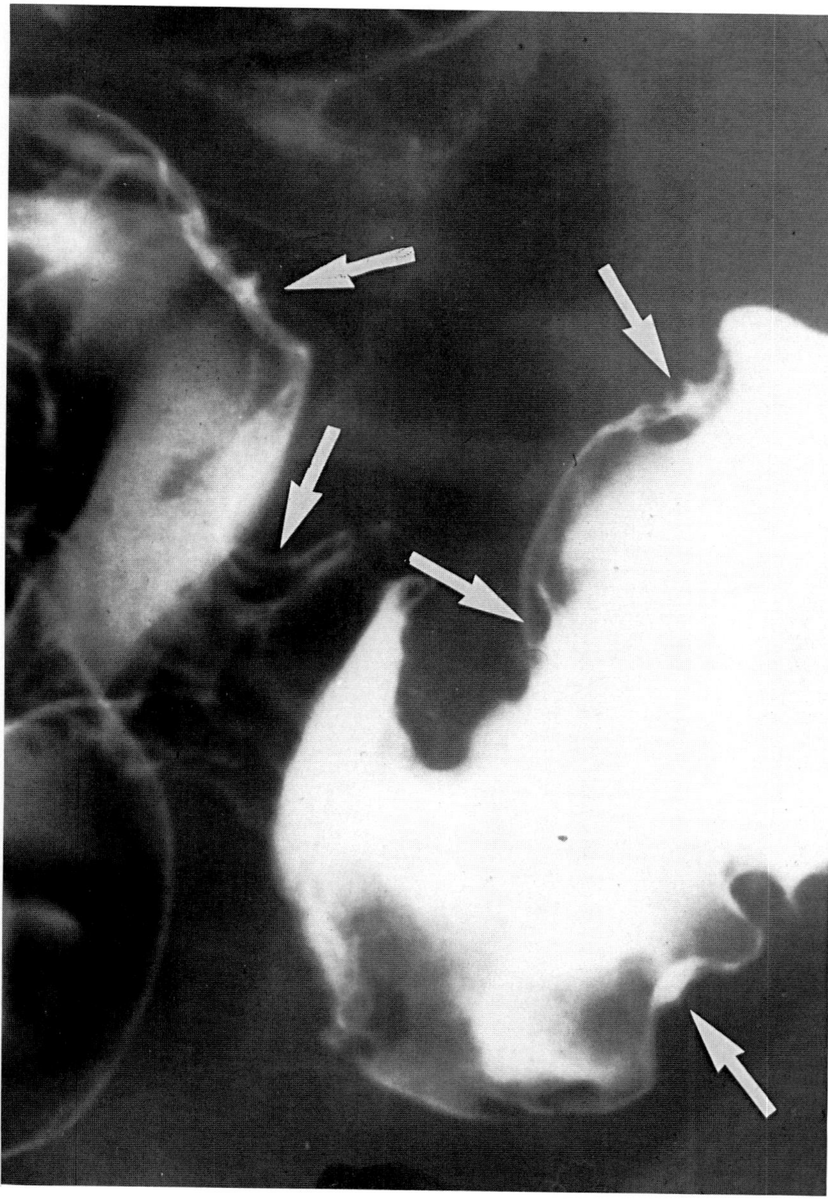

Figure 6 Advanced rectal Kaposi's sarcoma. Tumor nodules of advanced AIDS-related Kaposi's sarcoma (arrows) are seen on double-contrast barium examination of the rectosigmoid colon. (Reproduced from Reference 14 with permission.)

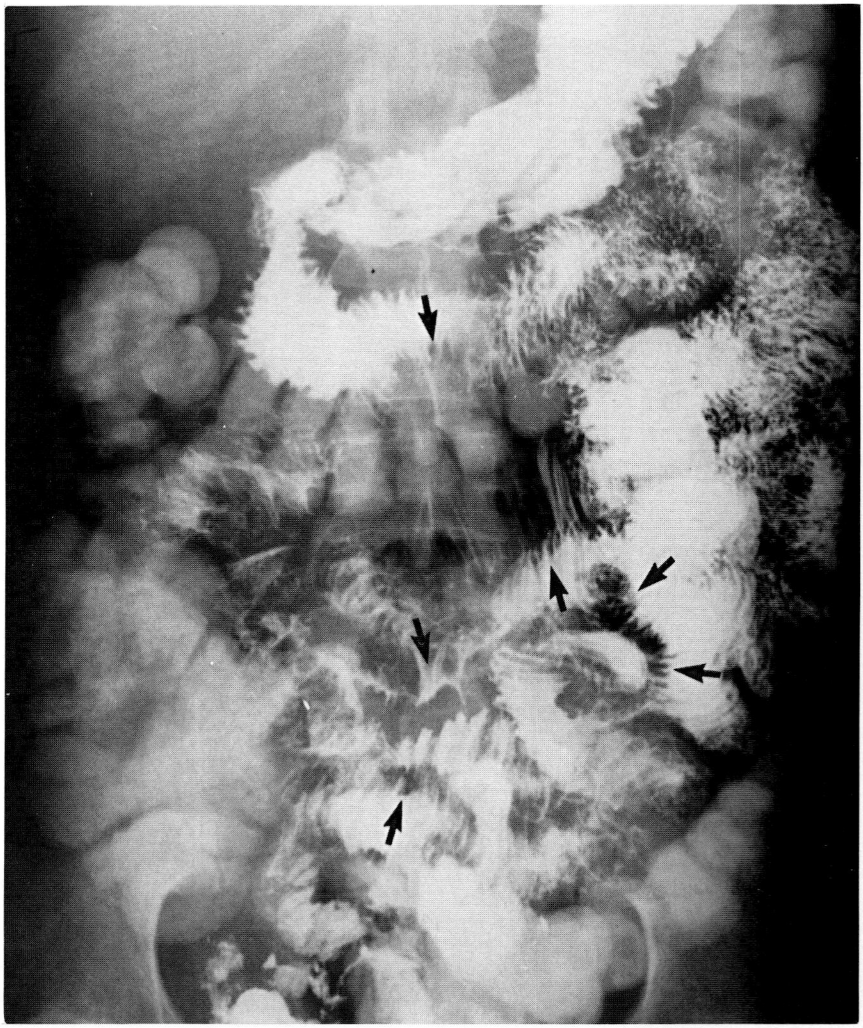

Figure 7 Small bowel Kaposi's sarcoma. Barium examination of the small bowel demonstrates diffuse thickening (arrows) of jejunal folds due to Kaposi's sarcoma.

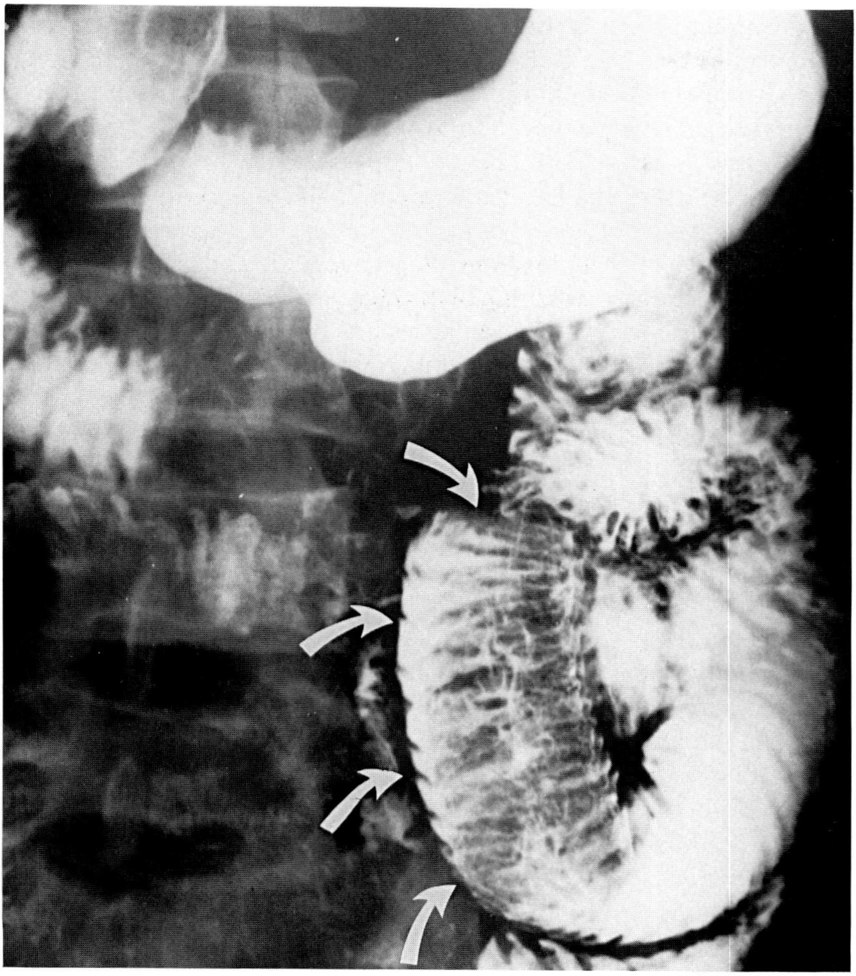

Figure 8 Kaposi's sarcoma and small bowel intussusception. Barium radiography of the small bowel demonstrates jejunojejunal intussusception (arrows) due to a tumor nodule of Kaposi's sarcoma.

and should be considered when diarrhea is present and increased small bowel secretions are seen on the radiographs (13). Moreover, opportunistic infection of the small bowel may be coexistent with Kaposi's sarcoma. However, focal areas of nodular masses are most suggestive of Kaposi's sarcoma (7,8,14).

Kaposi's sarcoma frequently involves the oral cavity, and even early lesions in the oral cavity and hypopharynx can be symptomatic because of their location. Pharyngography, that is, double-contrast barium examination of the pharynx and hypopharynx, can demonstrate the typical nodular lesions of symptomatic Kaposi's sarcoma (Figure 9) (13). It is helpful in the diagnostic evaluation of patients with AIDS who have dysphagia or odynophagia. It can demonstrate not only the tumor nodules or masses of Kaposi's sarcoma but also can localize the radiation port when local radiotherapy is indicated for palliation and improved quality of life. Pharyngography can serve as a useful screening study in patients with AIDS who have symptoms referrable to the hypopharynx and may be preferable to laryngoscopy for several reasons (15). Barium pharyngography sometimes can determine the full extent of disease better than direct visual examination because bulky lesions preclude complete evaluation at laryngoscopy. Compared with indirect laryngoscopy, barium pharyngography requires neither the operating room nor general anesthesia, it is less expensive, and it is more easily tolerated by the patient. Laryngoscopy is a more invasive procedure, and there is more risk to the examiner of exposure to the patient's body fluids. Concurrent evaluation of the upper gastrointestinal tract for possible multifocal disease can be performed readily with pharyngography. Additionally, computed tomography (CT) of the neck in patients with hypopharyngeal Kaposi's sarcoma may demonstrate invasion into adjacent soft tissues and lymph nodes (Figure 10) (15).

Radiographically, it may be difficult to differentiate Kaposi's sarcoma from non-Hodgkin's lymphoma in patients with AIDS, especially in the gastrointestinal tract. Lymphoma also may cause nodular masses and small bowel fold thickening. Moreover, these

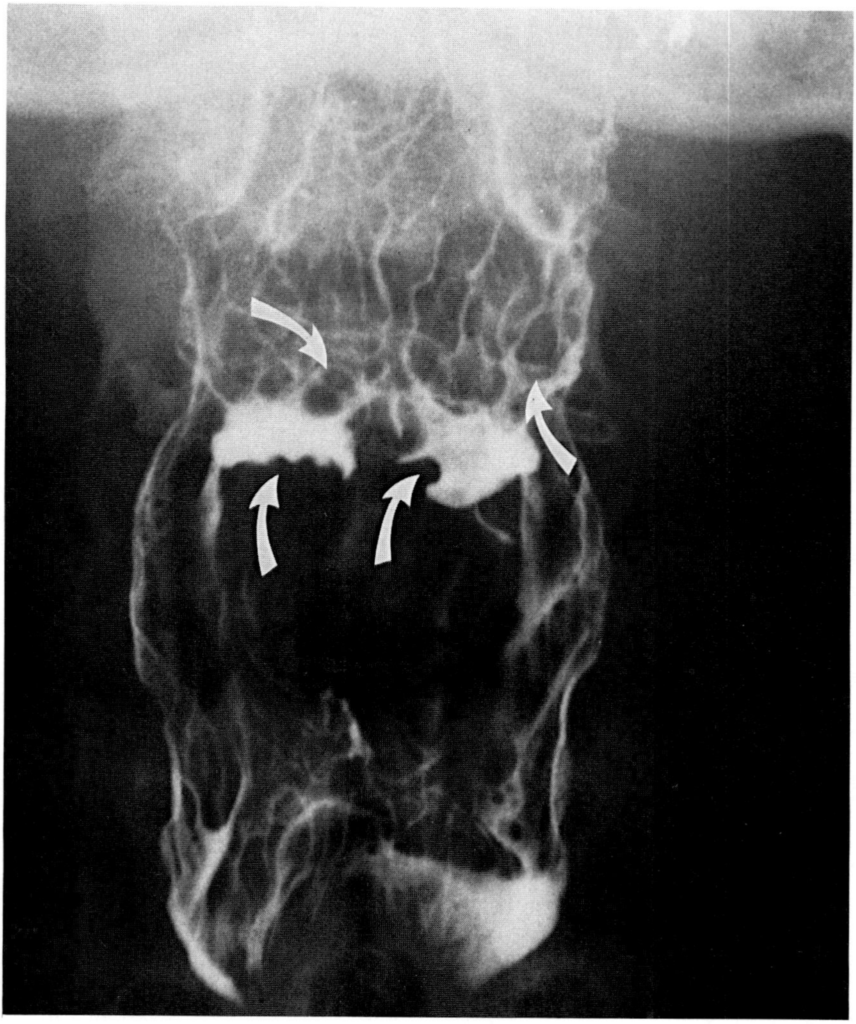

Figure 9A Hypopharyngeal Kaposi's sarcoma. Multiple small, but confluent nodules (arrows) of Kaposi's sarcoma are seen in the oropharynx and hypopharynx with deformity of the barium-filled valleculae, right greater than left.

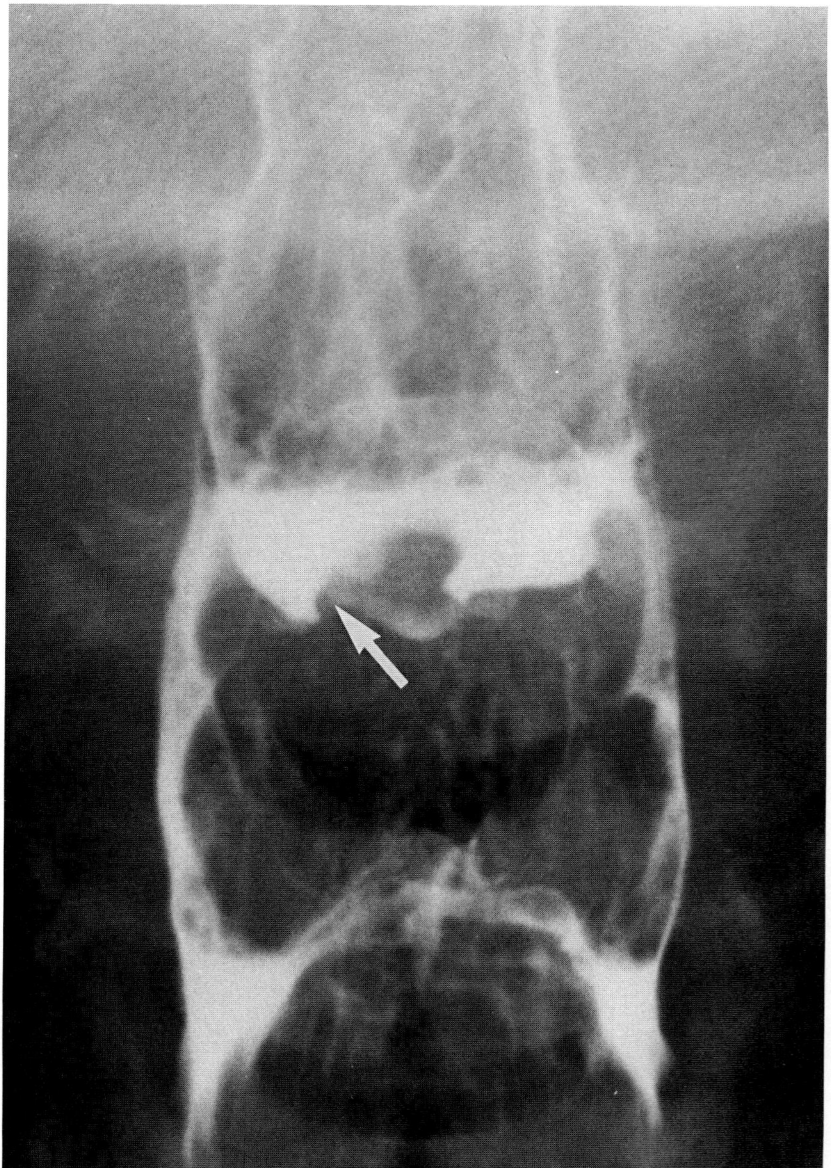

Figure 9B Reevaluation 10 months later, following local radiation therapy, demonstrates marked resolution of disease with minor residua of tumor nodularity causing a filling defect in right vallecula (arrow).

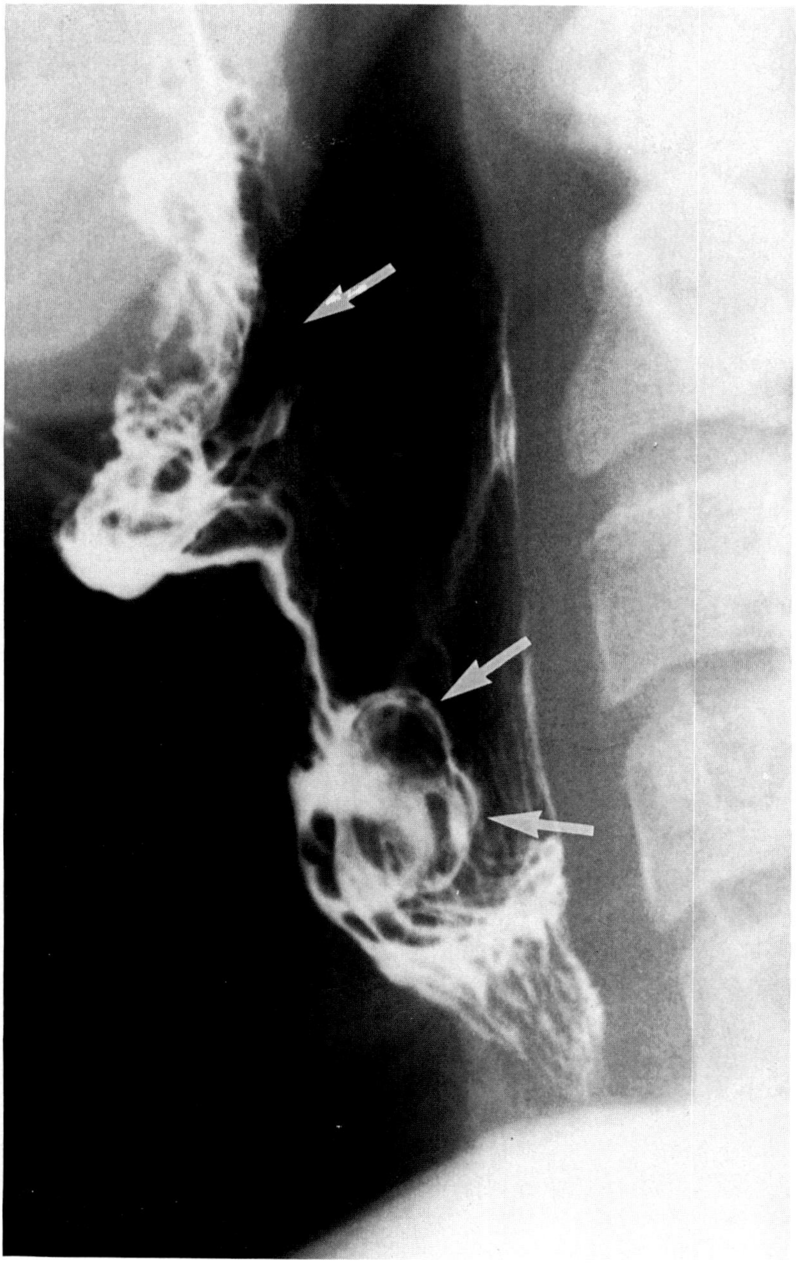

Figure 9C More extensive disease is seen in another patient whose lateral image on barium pharyngography demonstrates large nodular masses (arrows) of Kaposi's sarcoma in the left pyriform fossa, anterior wall of the hypopharynx, and base of the tongue. (Reproduced from Reference 15 with permission.)

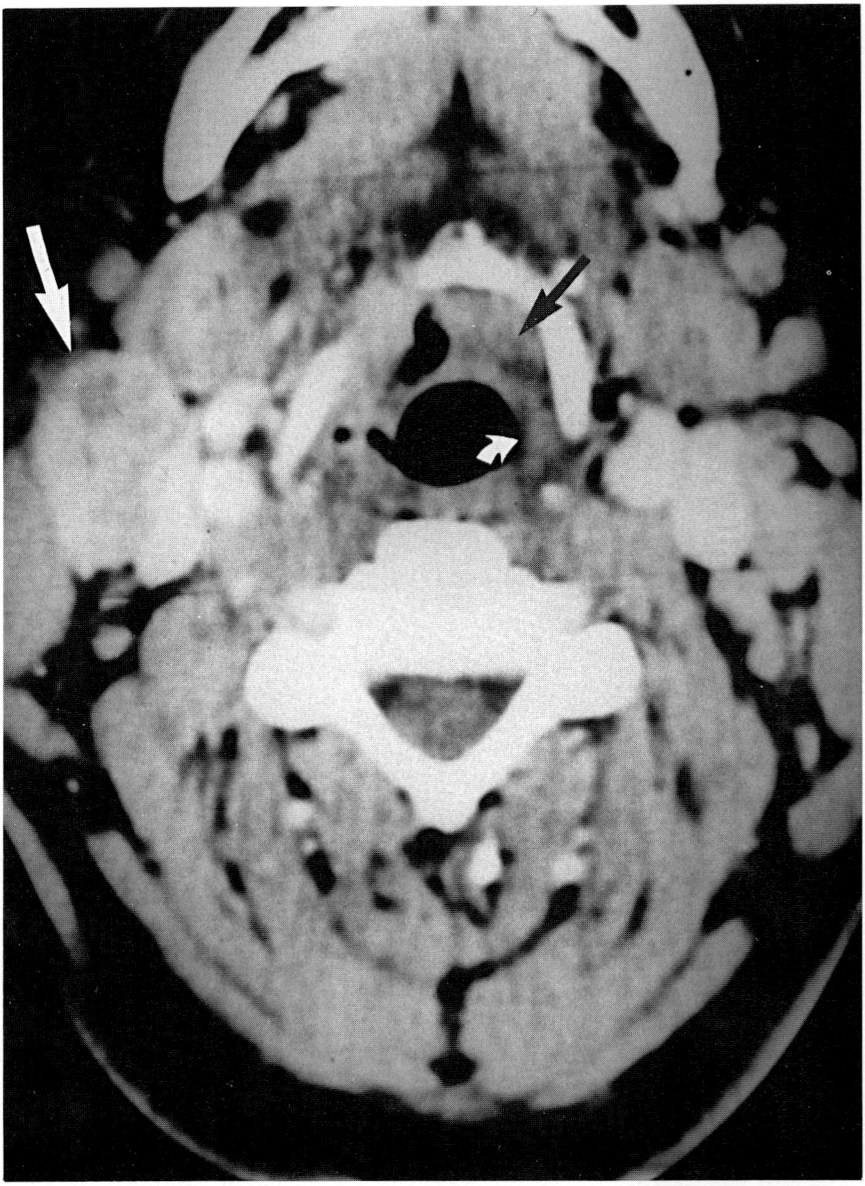

Figure 10A Kaposi's sarcoma of the neck. Computed tomography of the neck of a 31-year-old homosexual man demonstrates a large anterior cervical lymph node (straight white arrow) with focal areas of low attenuation, biopsy proven to be due to Kaposi's sarcoma. Note also Kaposi's sarcoma causing obliteration of the left vallecula (straight black arrow) and orifice of the left pyriform sinus (curved white arrow).

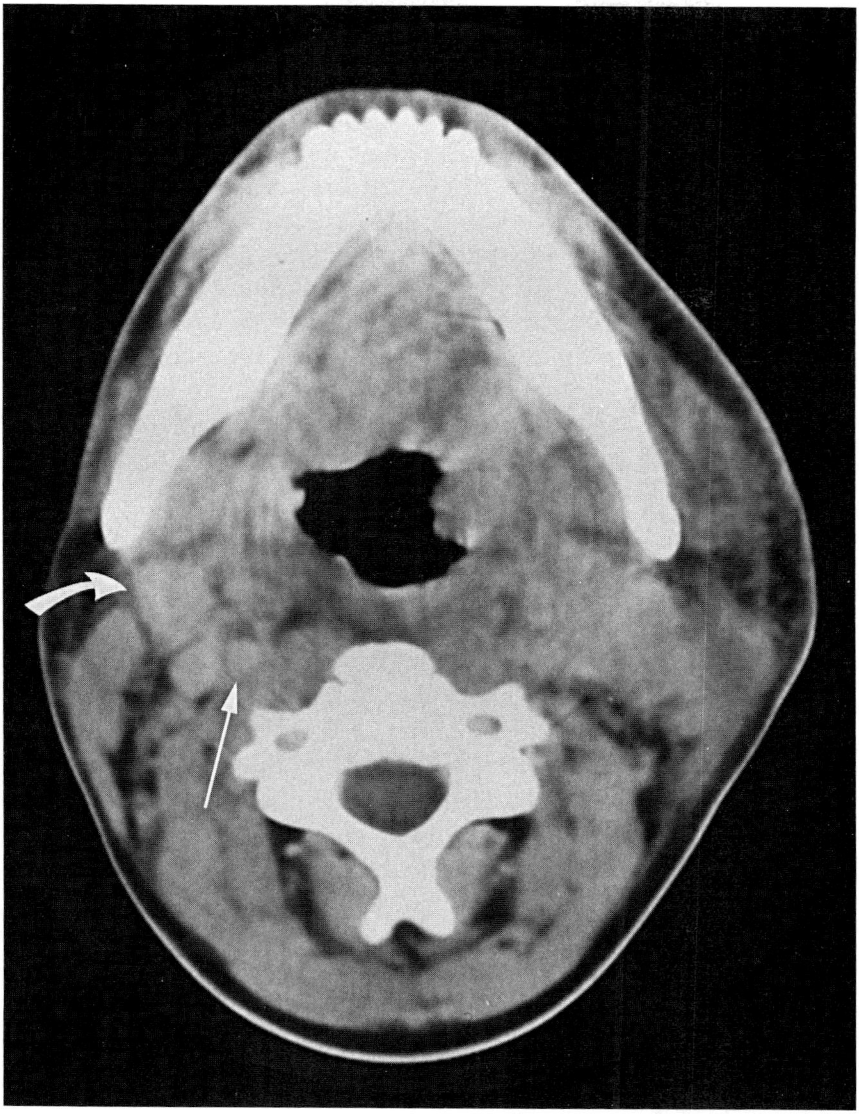

Figure 10B Computed tomographic image of a 22-year-old homosexual man with Kaposi's sarcoma demonstrates tumor infiltration of the parapharyngeal spaces bilaterally. Tumor surrounds the left carotid sheath and extends into the sternocleidomastoid muscle and the ill-defined but enlarged submandibular gland. Curved arrow indicates right submandibular gland; straight arrow indicates right carotid artery. (Reproduced from Reference 15 with permission.)

malignancies have been noted to coexist (9), sometimes in the same area, as in one patient who had focal lesions of each tumor in the duodenum (Figure 11). Lymphoma in patients with AIDS has an unusual propensity for extranodal sites of involvement compared with non-AIDS patients (16). Hence, it is important to recall that the radiographic differential of gastrointestinal thickening in patients with AIDS includes lymphoma as well as Kaposi's sarcoma and opportunistic infection.

Multifocal gastrointestinal abnormalities, that is, focal lesions in three or more sites, have been seen in 65–70% of homosexual AIDS patients who are referred for barium examination (9). The duodenum is the site most frequently abnormal in these patients, usually because of Kaposi's sarcoma or cryptosporidiosis. Both can cause fold thickening; nodularity is uncommon in the latter. Kaposi's sarcoma may be asymptomatic; cryptosporidiosis usually causes diarrhea. The multiplicity of sites of radiographic abnormality often is caused by multiple foci of Kaposi's sarcoma. Other causes of multifocal lesions include Kaposi's sarcoma and coexistent opportunistic infection (Figure 12), Kaposi's sarcoma and coexistent lymphoma (Figure 11), widely distributed opportunistic infection, and multiple opportunistic infections. In non-AIDS patients, the differential diagnosis of diseases that cause radiographic abnormalities in multiple sites of the gastrointestinal tract also includes Crohn's disease and lymphoma, neither of which commonly involves the duodenum. Hence, it has been suggested that the presence of multifocal gastrointestinal abnormalities, especially when the duodenum is involved, should suggest the diagnosis of AIDS even in patients not thought to be at high risk, and that Kaposi's sarcoma should be considered (9).

Abdominal Computed Tomography

Abnormalities on abdominal CT of homosexual men with Kaposi's sarcoma and AIDS are extremely common, but they are not diagnostic of tumor. Two-thirds of such patients have splenomegaly and abdominal lymphadenopathy, and more than 80% have rectal

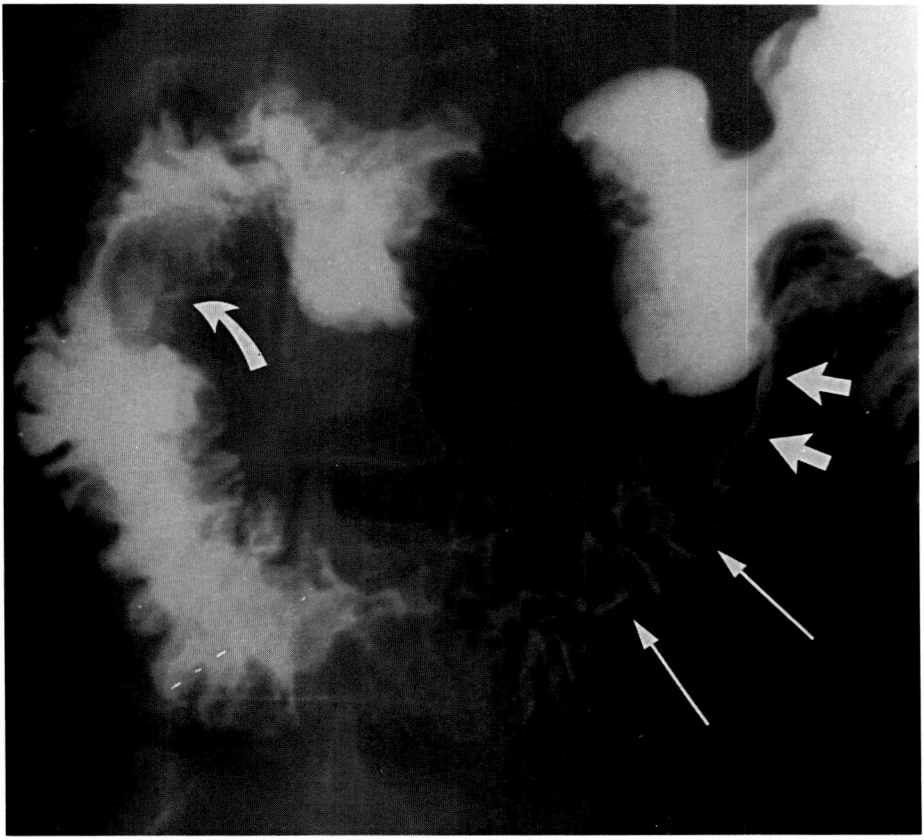

A

Figure 11 Coexistent malignancies. (A) Barium examination demonstrates nodular mass with central ulceration in the postbulbar duodenum (curved arrow); endoscopy diagnosed Kaposi's sarcoma. Irregular fold thickening (straight arrows) and mass causing concentric narrowing of the lumen of the transverse duodenum (arrowheads) was biopsy proven to be non-Hodgkin's Burkitt's-like lymphoma. (Reproduced from References 9 and 14 with permission.) (B) Computed tomographic scan corresponding to anatomic level shown in (A) demonstrates Kaposi's sarcoma mass (white arrow) displacing intraluminal contrast in proximal duodenum; note also the wall thickening of the distal transverse duodenum and luminal narrowing due to non-Hodgkin's lymphoma (black arrows). (Reproduced from Reference 9 with permission.) (C) Lymphangiogram demonstrates "foamy" appearance to enlarged lymph nodes caused by lymphoma and focal defects (arrows) of coexistent Kaposi's sarcoma.

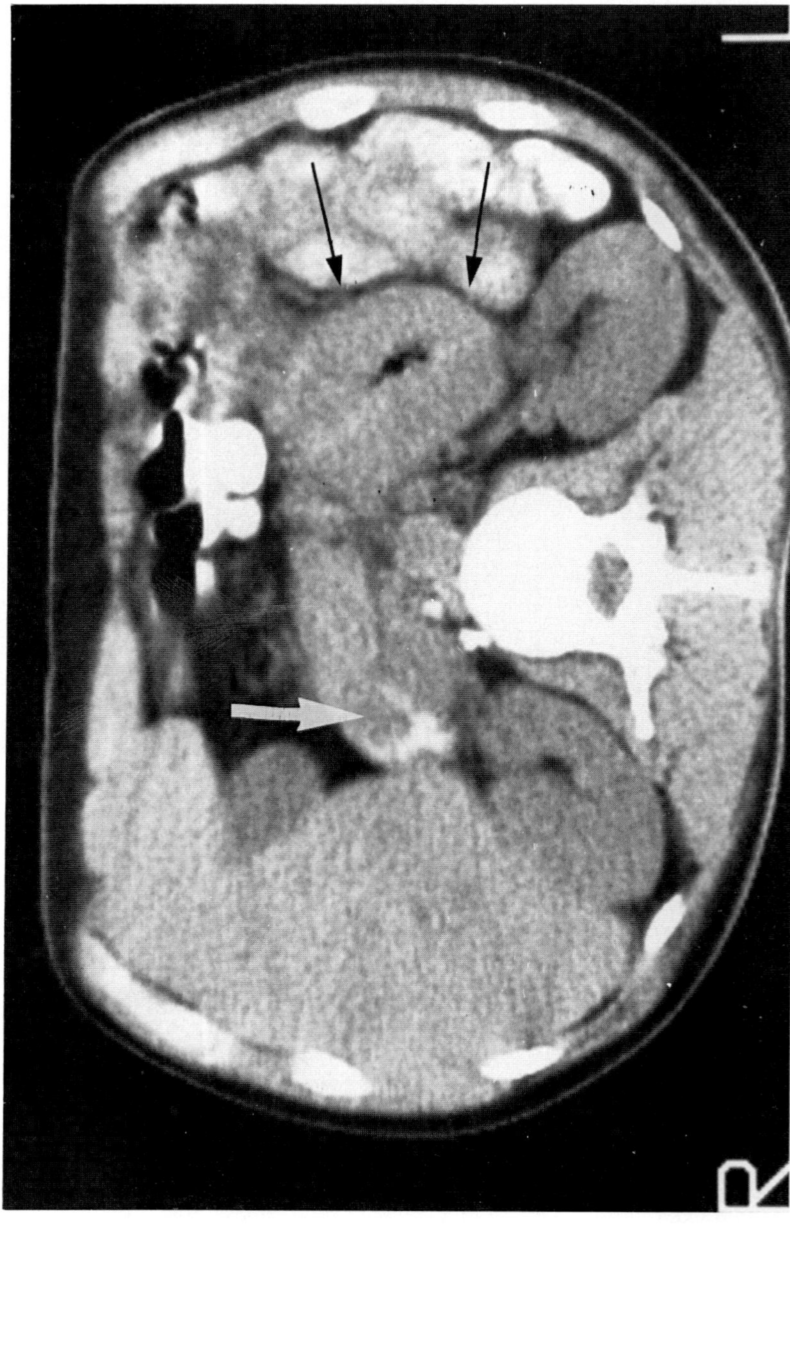

Figure 11B

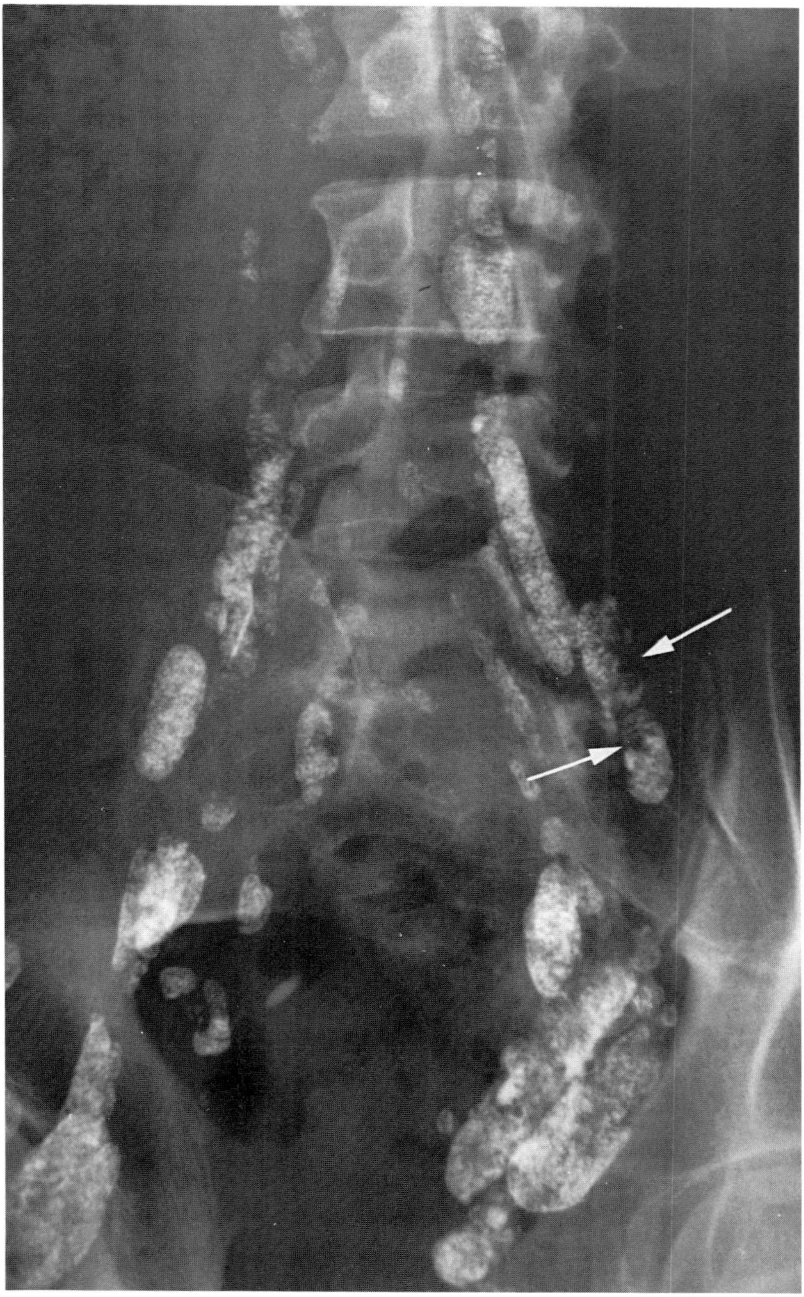

Figure 11C

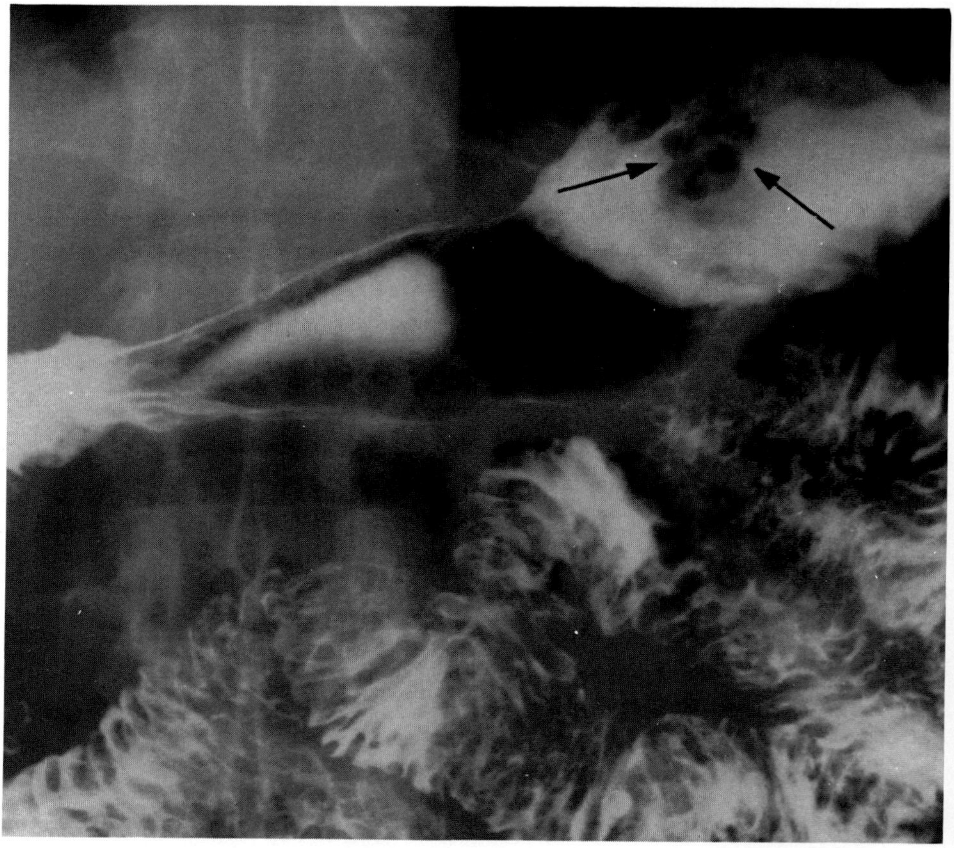

Figure 12 Multifocal gastrointestinal abnormalities. Nodular filling defects in the gastric fundus (arrows) were due to Kaposi's sarcoma in this homosexual man with AIDS. Both cytomegalovirus and cryptosporidium were present in the gastric antrum (nondistensible) and in the small bowel (thick folds). (Reproduced from References 9 and 14 with permission.)

wall thickening (17). However, these findings are also seen as a typical triad of abnormalities noted on abdominal CT in homosexual men with AIDS-related complex (ARC). CT findings that are supplementary to this triad suggest AIDS and possible intra-abdominal Kaposi's sarcoma. They are discussed below and are compared with those findings associated with ARC and those of AIDS with lymphoma and/or disseminated infection.

Kaposi's sarcoma is uncommonly seen in the liver or spleen in patients with AIDS, but when present, it appears as focal areas of low density (18). Percutaneous fine-needle aspiration biopsy is necessary in order to differentiate Kaposi's sarcoma lesions from lymphoma or infection. Splenomegaly is more often accompanied by hepatomegaly in patients with AIDS (with or without Kaposi's sarcoma) than ARC, but both the liver and spleen are of normal density and are homogeneous throughout in ARC. Focal hepatic or splenic lesions are not seen in ARC, and their presence suggests tumor or infection.

The rectal or perirectal abnormalities in homosexual men with ARC include thickening of the rectal wall and increased attenuation of the perirectal fat (Figure 13) (17). Such findings in these patients, who are often asymptomatic at the time of the CT examination, are thought to be caused by repeated episodes of proctitis due to venereal infections (19). However, the rectal thickening cannot be differentiated from the CT findings of Kaposi's sarcoma involving the rectum (17), although asymmetric thickening would suggest the latter (Figure 14) (14). When Kaposi's sarcoma is suspected, proctosigmoidoscopy or colonoscopy is diagnostic.

Abdominal lymphadenopathy, even in the presence of known skin or peripheral nodal Kaposi's sarcoma, does not necessarily indicate widespread involvement with Kaposi's sarcoma (17). It is important to emphasize that the lymphadenopathy seen in AIDS-related complex is a characteristic pattern of clusters of normal sized to mildly enlarged lymph nodes (0.5–1.0 cm), which are present in abnormally increased numbers (Figure 15) (17). They are seen throughout the mesentery, retroperitoneum, and pelvic chains. CT-guided percutaneous fine-needle aspiration of enlarged

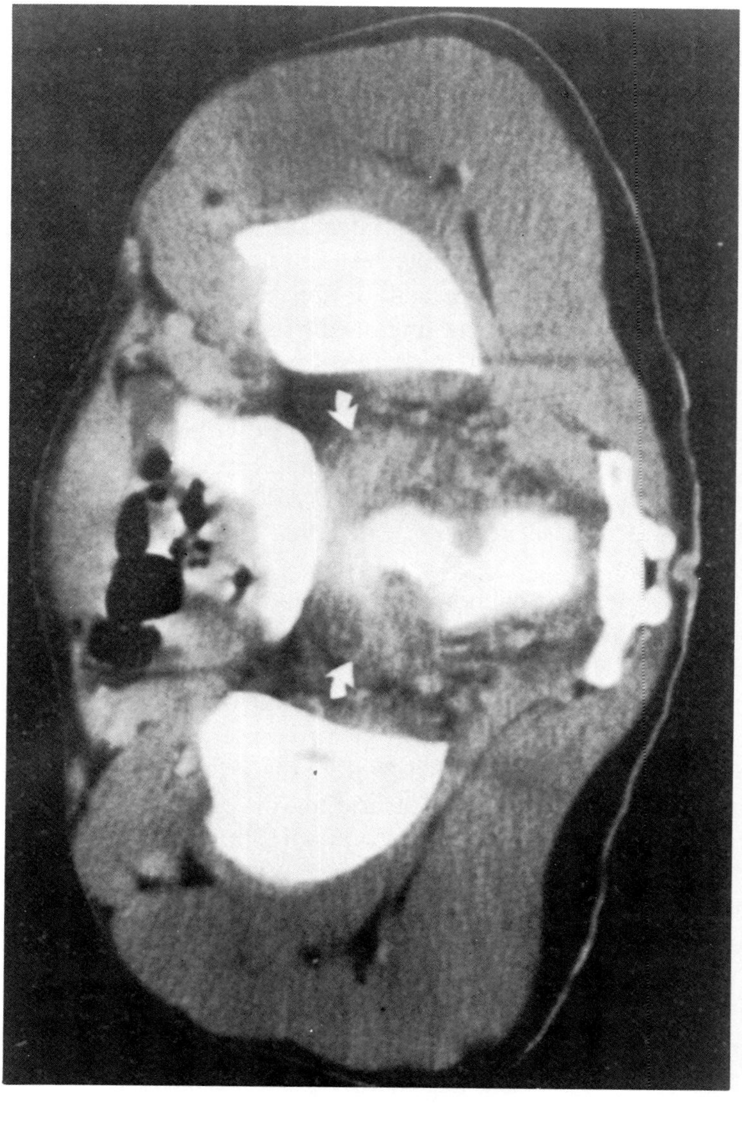

Figure 13 AIDS-related complex (ARC) with perirectal inflammation. CT demonstrates symmetrical thickening of the wall of the rectosigmoid colon and diffuse infiltration of the perirectal fat (arrows), which is abnormally dense. (Reproduced from Reference 18 with permission.)

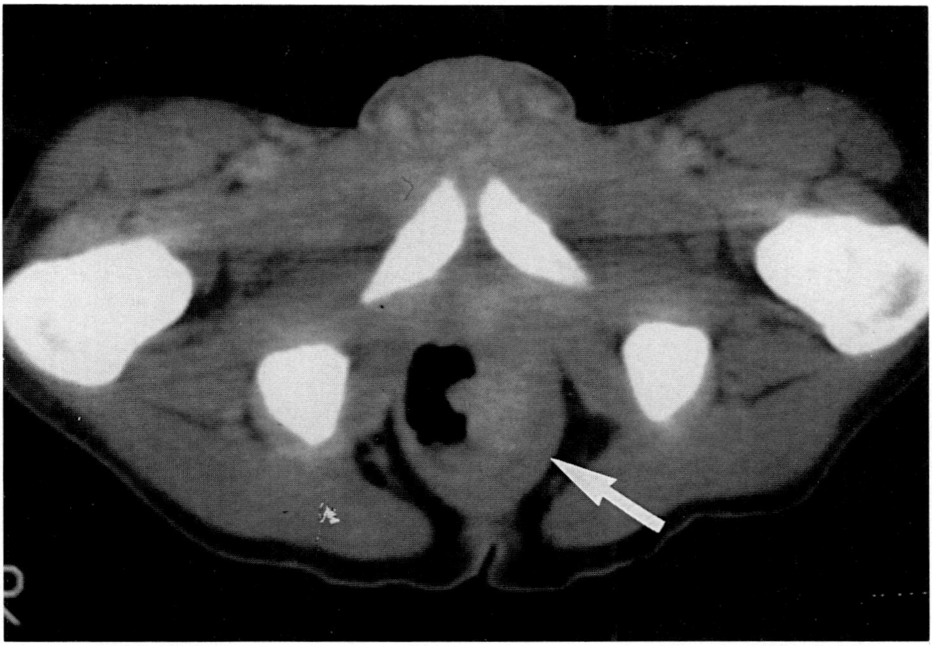

Figure 14 Rectal Kaposi's sarcoma. CT of patient with AIDS and rectal Kaposi's sarcoma demonstrates asymmetric thickening of the rectal wall (arrow). (Reproduced from Reference 14 with permission.)

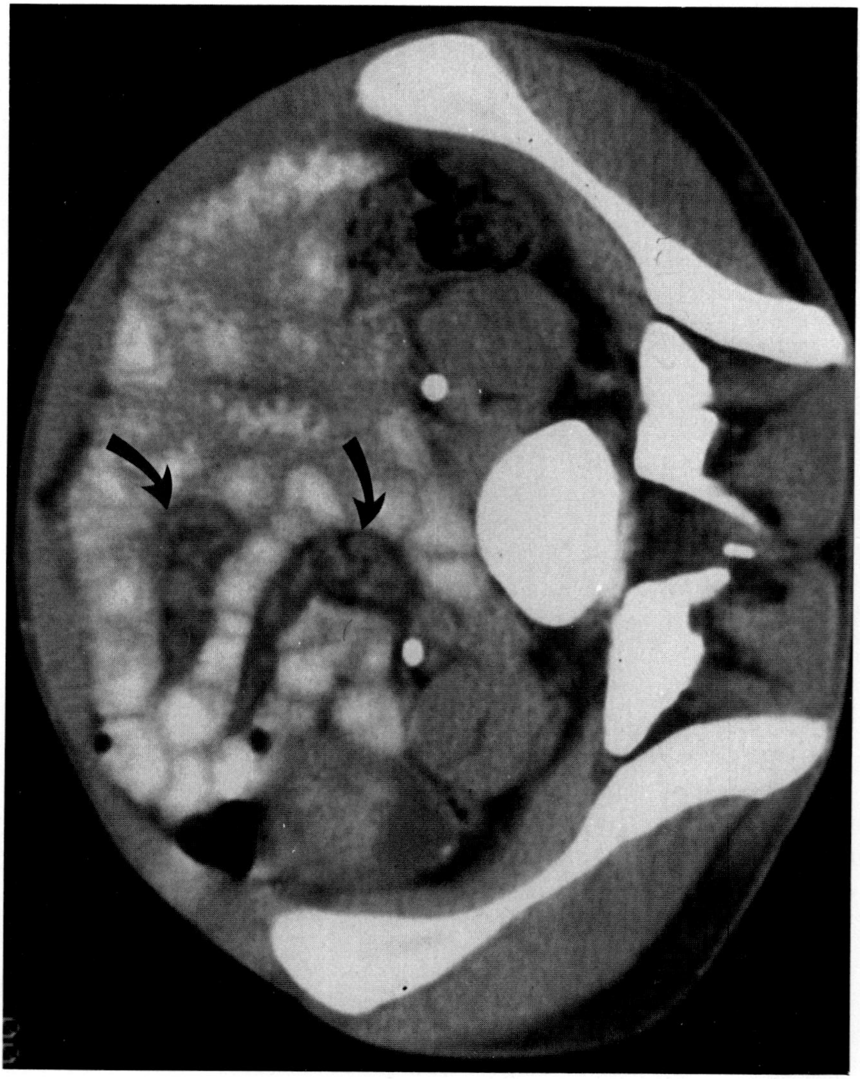

Figure 15 Mesenteric lymphadenopathy of ARC. Typical clusters of small lymph nodes are present throughout the small bowel mesentery (arrows).

lymph nodes usually reveals reactive hyperplasia, and this procedure generally is no longer performed when the characteristic radiographic pattern is present.

In contradistinction, the homosexual patient with bulky (>1.0–1.5 cm) abdominal lymphadenopathy (Figure 16) is more likely to have AIDS than the AIDS-related complex, and the nodal enlargement usually is due to lymphoma, Kaposi's sarcoma, or infection with *Mycobacterium avium-intracellulare* (MAI) (18,20). Central low density on CT (Figure 10B) (or central low signal intensity on magnetic resonance imaging) (Figure 17) due to necrosis is seen occasionally in large nodes infiltrated with Kaposi's sarcoma or MAI. The radiographic findings are not specific for tumor or infection; CT-guided percutaneous fine-needle aspiration can be diagnostic. All aspirates should be stained for acid-fast bacilli and cultured for mycobacterium. The bulky lymphadenopathy in patients with disseminated MAI has been noted to be more prominent in the mesentery than the retroperitoneum (20). This finding may be related to the small bowel involvement with MAI, which in patients with AIDS can closely resemble Whipple's disease both radiographically and pathologically (21–23). The clinical and radiographic pattern of small bowel disease and mesenteric lymphadenopathy has suggested the intestine as a common portal of entry for MAI (21).

Kaposi's sarcoma can cause unusual abnormalities on abdominal computed tomography because of its propensity to involve virtually any organ in the body in patients with AIDS, especially late in the disease (Figure 18). Enlargement of any organ or soft tissue structure with associated low attenuation suggests possible tumor involvement (Figure 19). Adrenal masses have been seen as well as diffuse infiltration of intraperitoneal and retroperitoneal fat. Circumscribed lesions of homogeneous soft tissue density in subcutaneous fat of the abdominal wall are manifestations of extensive skin lesions. Focal or diffuse thickening of the wall of the gastrointestinal tract is noted readily on CT (Figure 20). Diffuse thickening cannot be differentiated radiographically from an infectious cause, but when thickening is focal and nodular, Kaposi's sarcoma should be suspected.

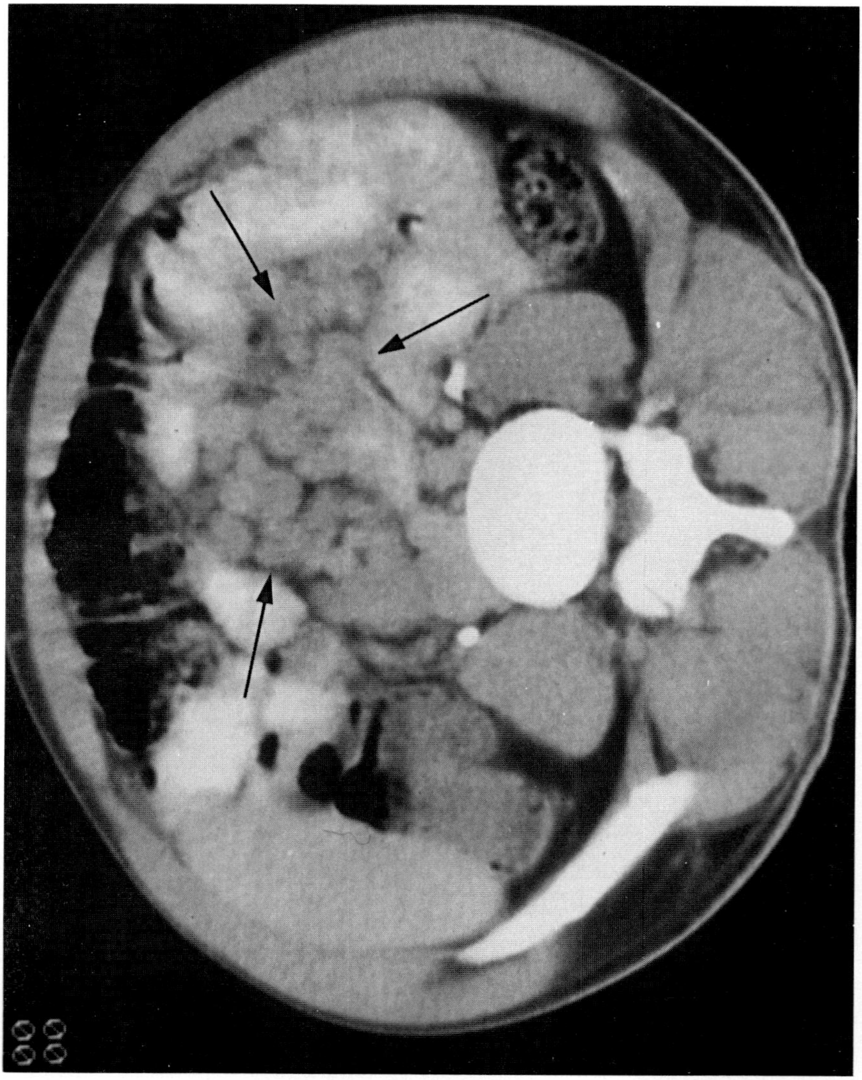

A

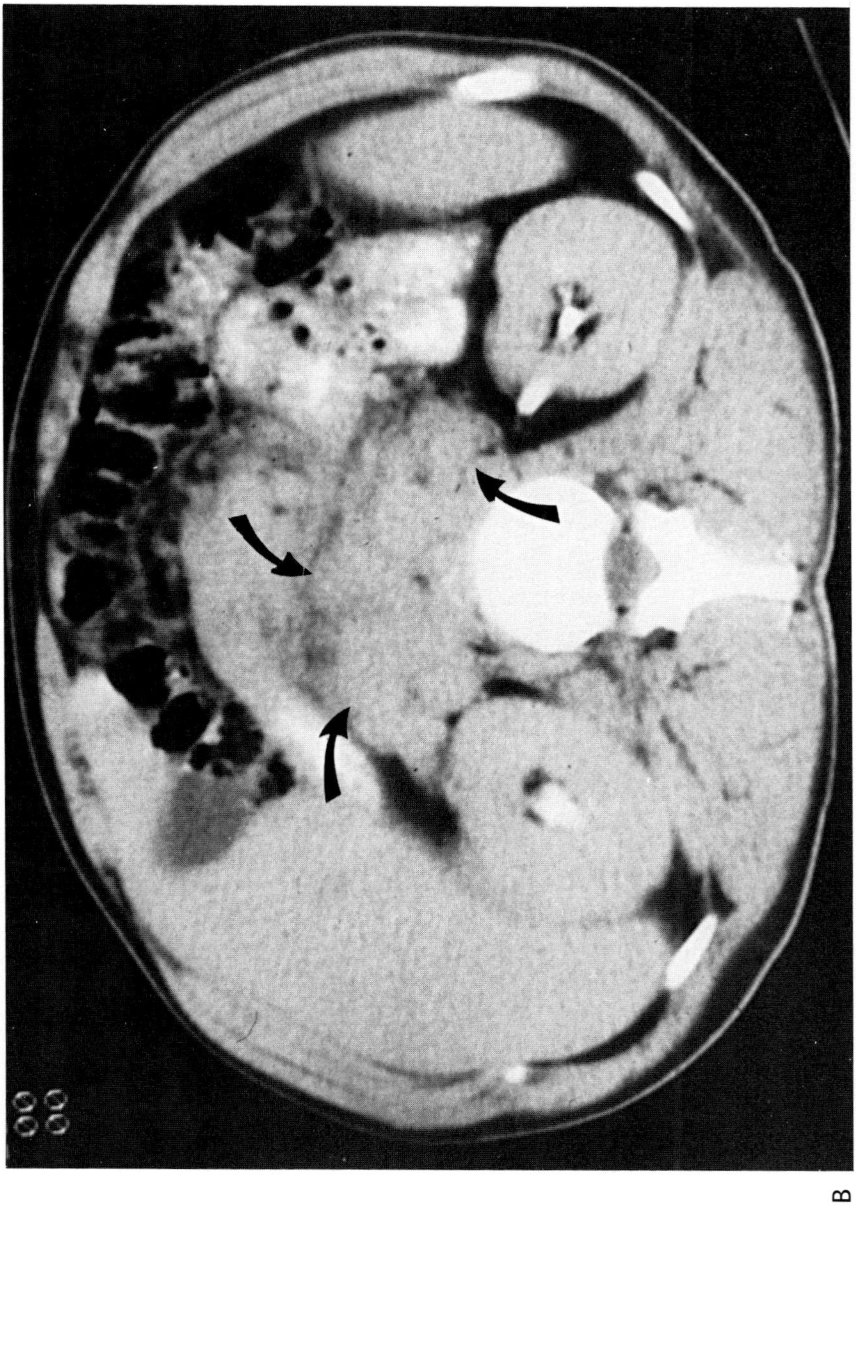

B

Figure 16 Lymphadenopathy of AIDS-related Kaposi's sarcoma. Large mesenteric (A) and retroperitoneal (B) lymph nodes (arrows) typical of those seen with Kaposi's sarcoma, MAI, or lymphoma in patients with AIDS. (Figure A reproduced from Reference 14 with permission.)

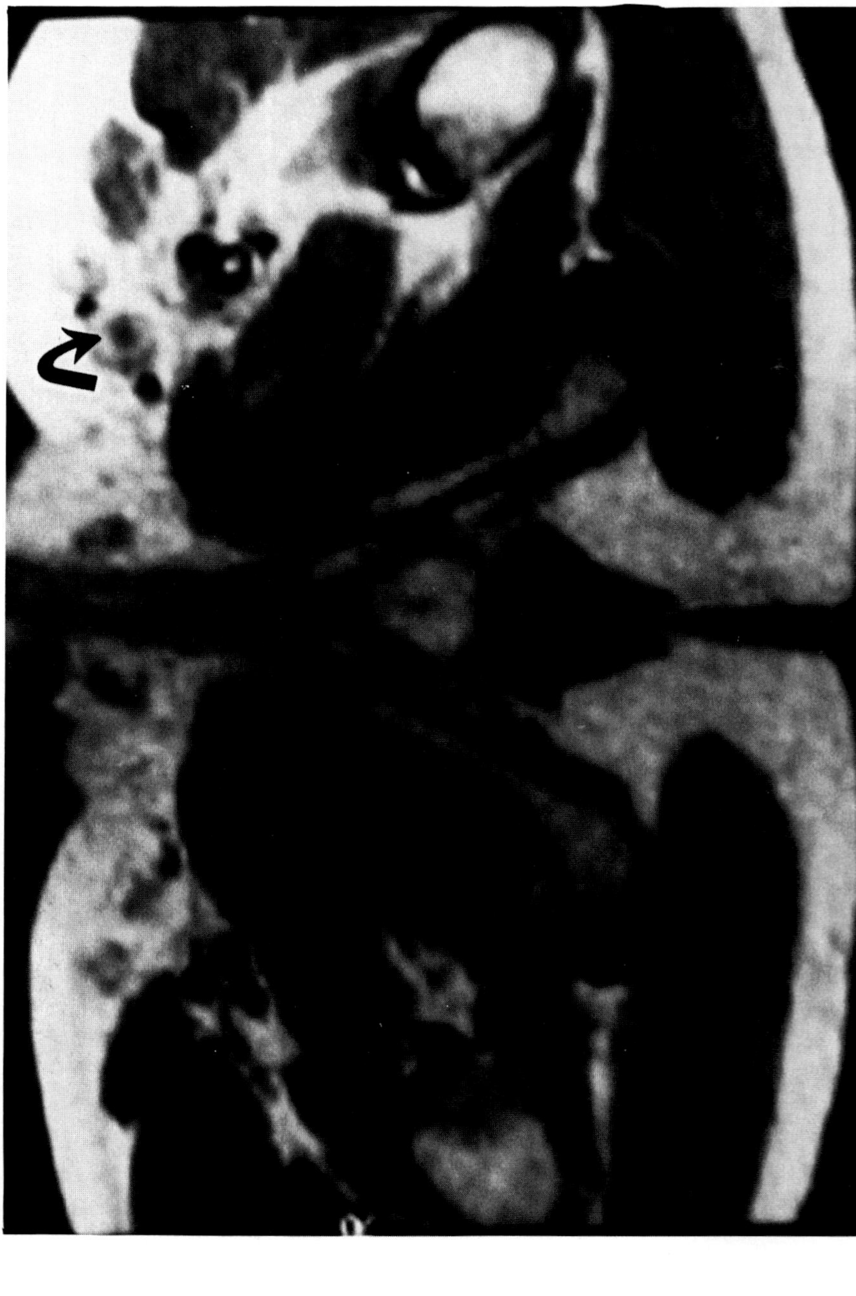

Figure 17A Inguinal lymphadenopathy. Magnetic resonance imaging demonstrates central low signal intensity (arrow) of inguinal lymphadenopathy; biopsy-demonstrated necrosis, and Kaposi's sarcoma.

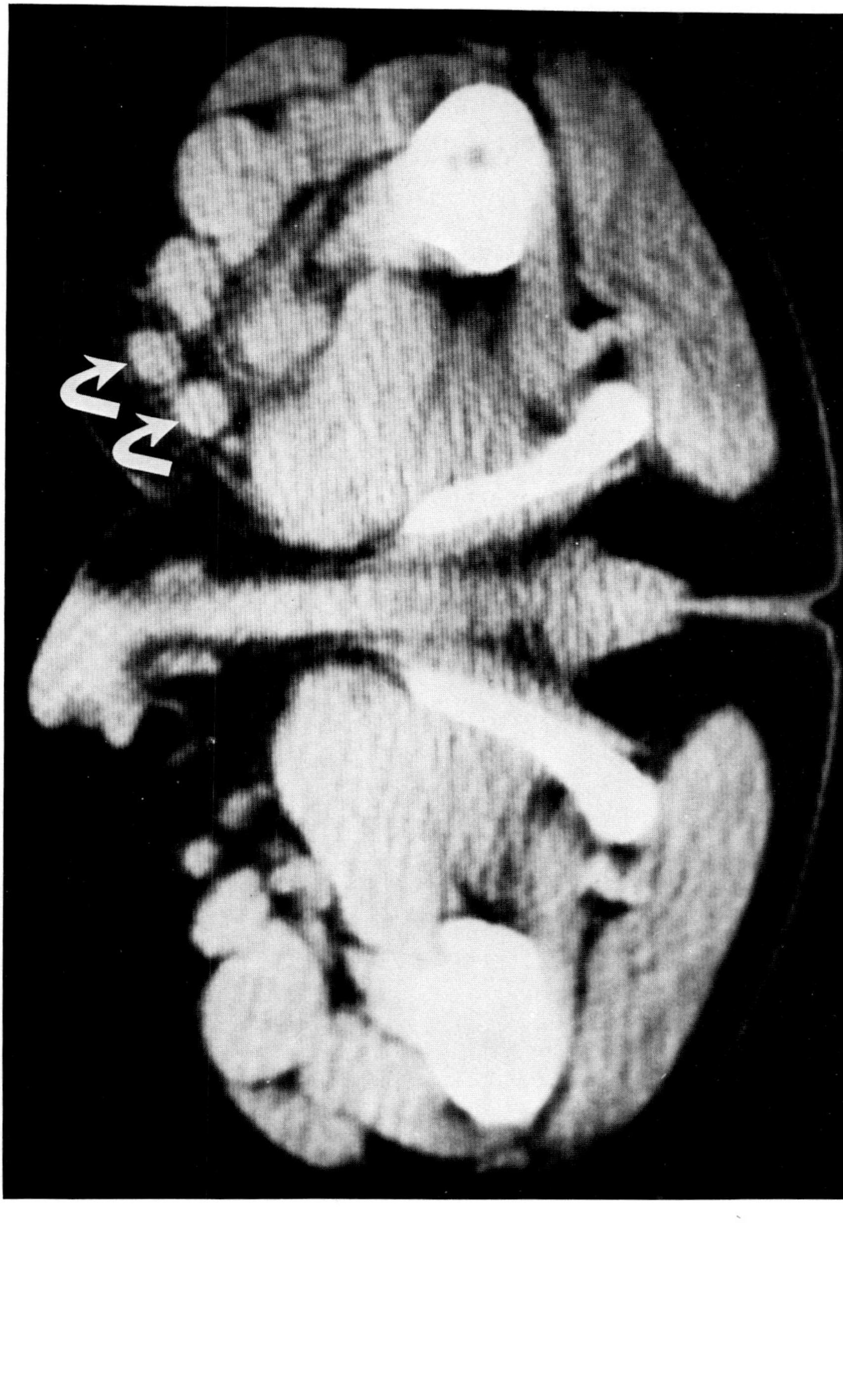

Figure 17B CT of the same patient shows enlarged inguinal nodes only (arrows); it does not demonstrate a low-density center.

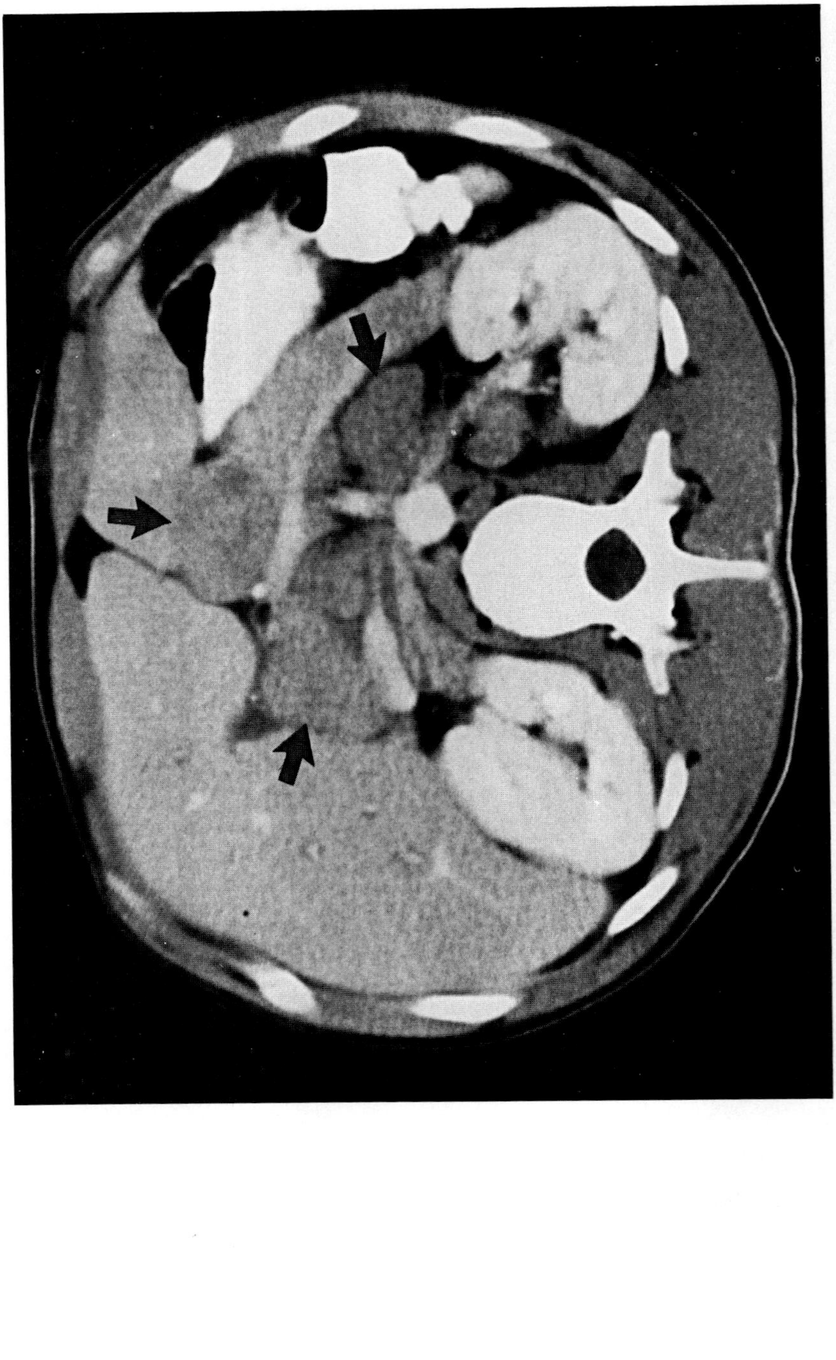

Figure 18 Lymphadenopathic form of Kaposi's sarcoma. CT of bulky retroperitoneal lymph nodes in the periportal and peripancreatic chains (arrows). (Reproduced from Reference 18 with permission.)

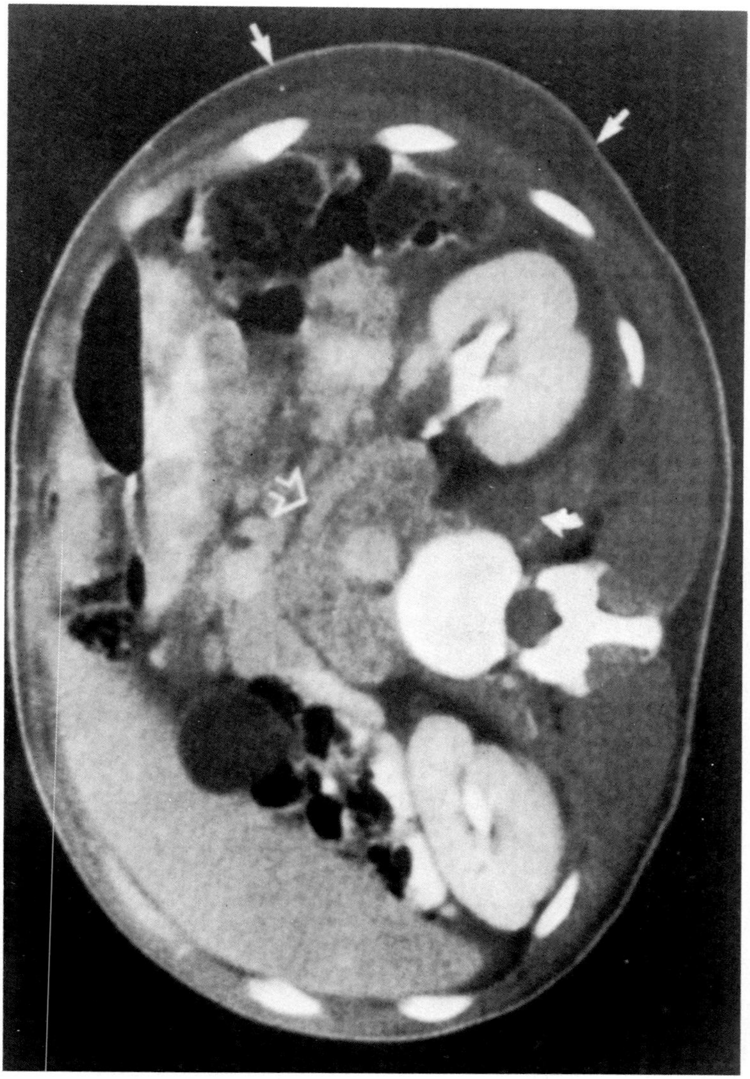

Figure 19 Widespread abdominal Kaposi's sarcoma. CT demonstrates extensive Kaposi's sarcoma involving para-aortic lymph nodes (open arrowhead), left psoas muscle (curved arrowhead), and left abdominal wall (straight arrowheads). (Reproduced from Reference 18 with permission.)

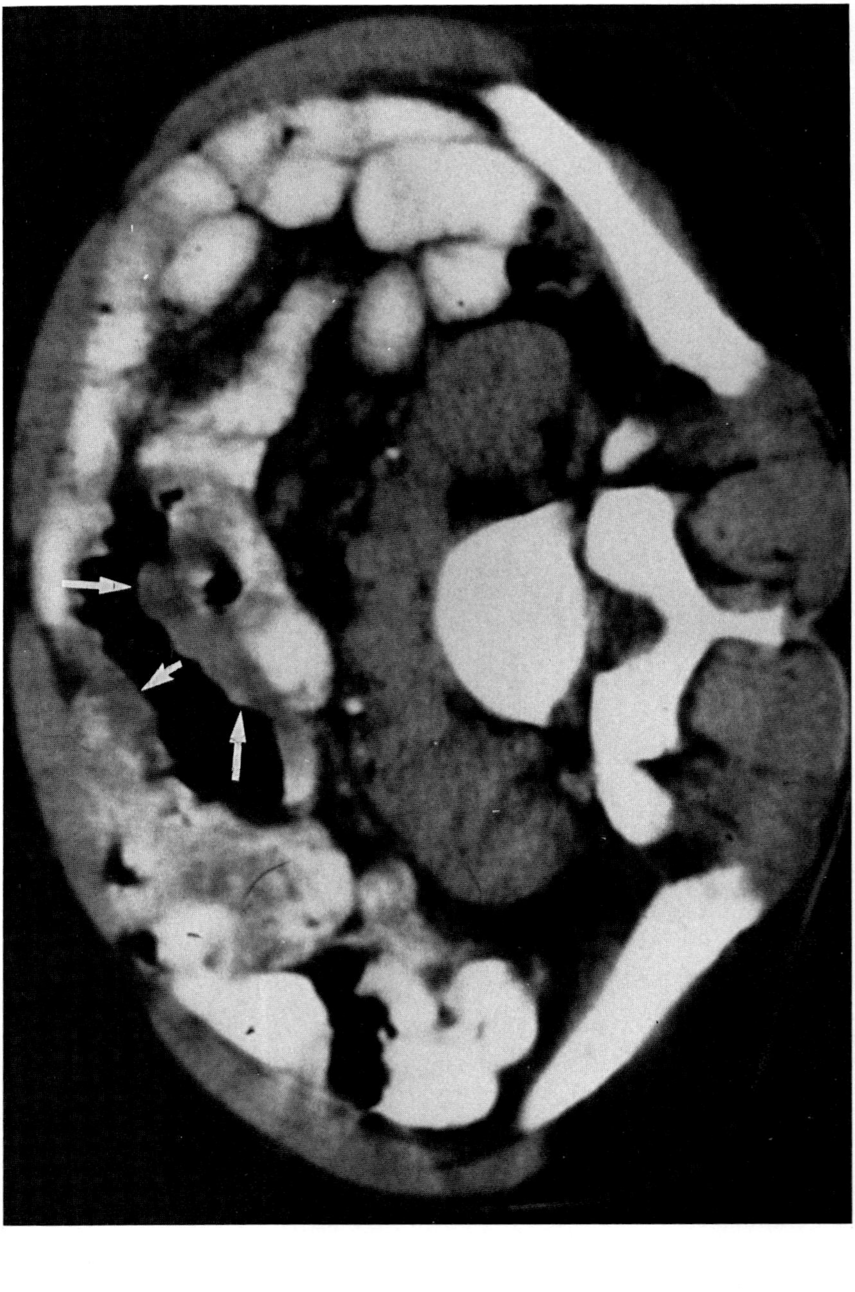

Figure 20 Small bowel Kaposi's sarcoma. Focal tumor nodules of Kaposi's sarcoma (arrows) protrude into the lumen of a segment of small bowel in this patient with AIDS.

CHEST RADIOGRAPHY: PLAIN CHEST RADIOGRAPH

Pulmonary Kaposi's sarcoma generally is seen late in the clinical course of AIDS. When present, it often is preterminal. It may be superimposed on opportunistic lung infection, or it may be isolated. Several chest radiographic findings suggest the presence of Kaposi's sarcoma, even in the setting of known opportunistic infection. Nodular lung densities (Figure 21) and linear infiltrates are commonly seen in pulmonary Kaposi's sarcoma (10,24–28) but are not typical of opportunistic lung infection alone (25,28,29). Also, pleural effusion (Figure 22) can be seen in patients with isolated *Pneumocystis carinii* pneumonia, but is more common in those with Kaposi's sarcoma, either alone or superimposed on *P. carinii* pneumonia (15,23,28). A change in the radiographic pattern of lung disease in a patient known to have *P. carinii* pneumonia or another opportunistic infection should prompt rebiopsy, especially when there is development of parenchymal nodules, linear infiltrates, pleural effusion, or mediastinal or hilar lymphadenopathy.

Isolated intrathoracic lymphadenopathy is not a helpful finding in the evaluation of possible pulmonary Kaposi's sarcoma. It is not seen in patients with isolated pulmonary Kaposi's sarcoma in the absence of extensive visceral and cutaneous disease but may be seen when coexistent intrathoracic lymphoma or opportunistic infection is present (30). In patients with known pulmonary Kaposi's sarcoma, intrathoracic lymphadenopathy cannot routinely be attributed to this neoplasm. With further evaluation, coexistent pulmonary infection generally will be found, usually implicating *P. carinii* pneumonia, tuberculosis, MAI, cryptococcus, or cytomegalovirus (30). However, in patients with ARC, mediastinal and/or hilar lymphadenopathy should not be considered to be due to benign reactive hyperplasia. Diagnostic evaluation should be performed and generally will disclose *P. carinii* pneumonia, another opportunistic infection, lymphoma, or Kaposi's sarcoma.

Positive radionuclide lung scans with gallium 67 are more suggestive of pulmonary infection than Kaposi's sarcoma. Diffuse

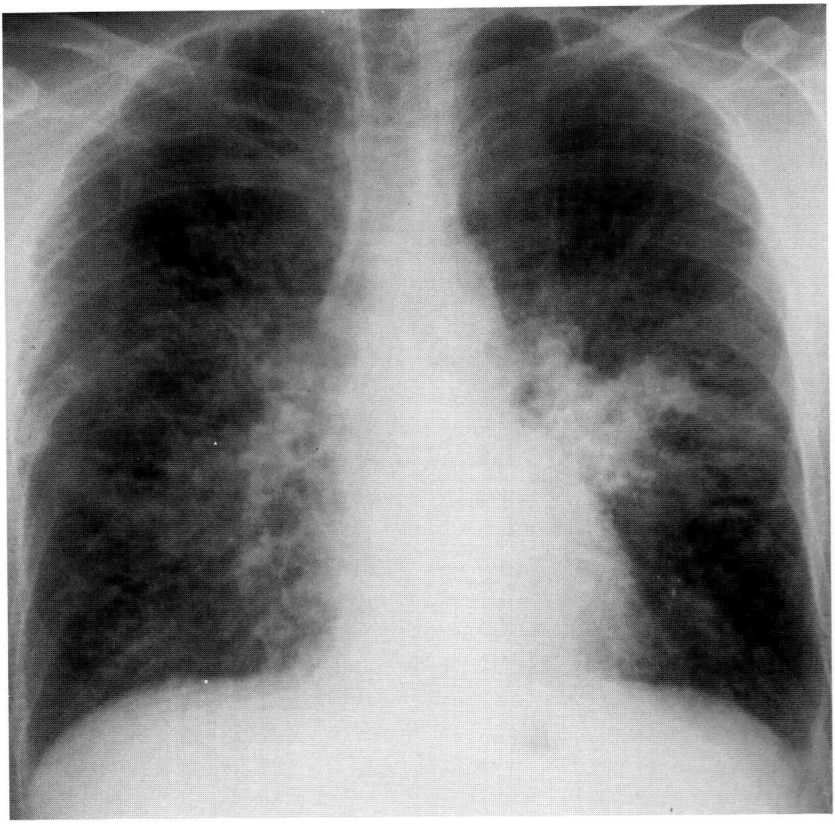

Figure 21 Lung Kaposi's sarcoma. Subtle nodular densities in the lung parenchyma of this patient with bilateral infiltrates and known *Pneumocystis carinii* pneumonia prompted rebiopsy, which was positive for Kaposi's sarcoma.

activity will be demonstrated throughout both lungs in 100% of patients with *P. carinii* pneumonia and in approximately 90% of patients with Kaposi's sarcoma and opportunistic infection. In contradistinction, only 30% of patients with pulmonary Kaposi's sarcoma alone have positive gallium scans.

A review of the radiographic presentation of *P. carinii* pneumonia (31–33) is helpful when considering pulmonary Kaposi's sarcoma. Patients with early pneumonia commonly have a normal chest radiograph. At this time gallium 67 uptake with radionuclide imaging will be increased throughout both lungs and bronchoscopic washings will be diagnostic. A high index of suspicion for *P. carinii* pneumonia shoud be raised when subtle interstitial changes are present on the chest radiograph. More advanced pneumonia will produce symmetrical, bilateral, homogenous infiltrates (24). With further progression, coalescent infiltrates demonstrate a uniform pattern similar to that in classic pulmonary edema, often with sparing of the peripheral lung.

INTRACEREBRAL KAPOSI'S SARCOMA

To date, there are two reports of cerebral Kaposi's sarcoma in patients with AIDS. One patient demonstrated a right frontal lesion on CT performed with intravenous contrast. The pathologically proven tumor appeared as a homogeneous, hyperdense lesion with little surrounding edema and little mass effect (Figure 23) (34). The second patient had a normal CT examination (Figure 24A) but demonstrated a homogeneous mass of high signal intensity on magnetic resonance imaging with a relatively T2 weighted sequence (TR = 1.5 sec, TE = 105 msec) (Figure 24B) (35). The findings are not specific for Kaposi's sarcoma on either imaging technique. Early infectious lesions have had a similar appearance on CT, although they are often hyperdense in the periphery. Similarly, focal areas of high-intensity signal on magnetic resonance can be seen with infection and with primary lymphoma of the brain. The usual appearance of primary central nervous system

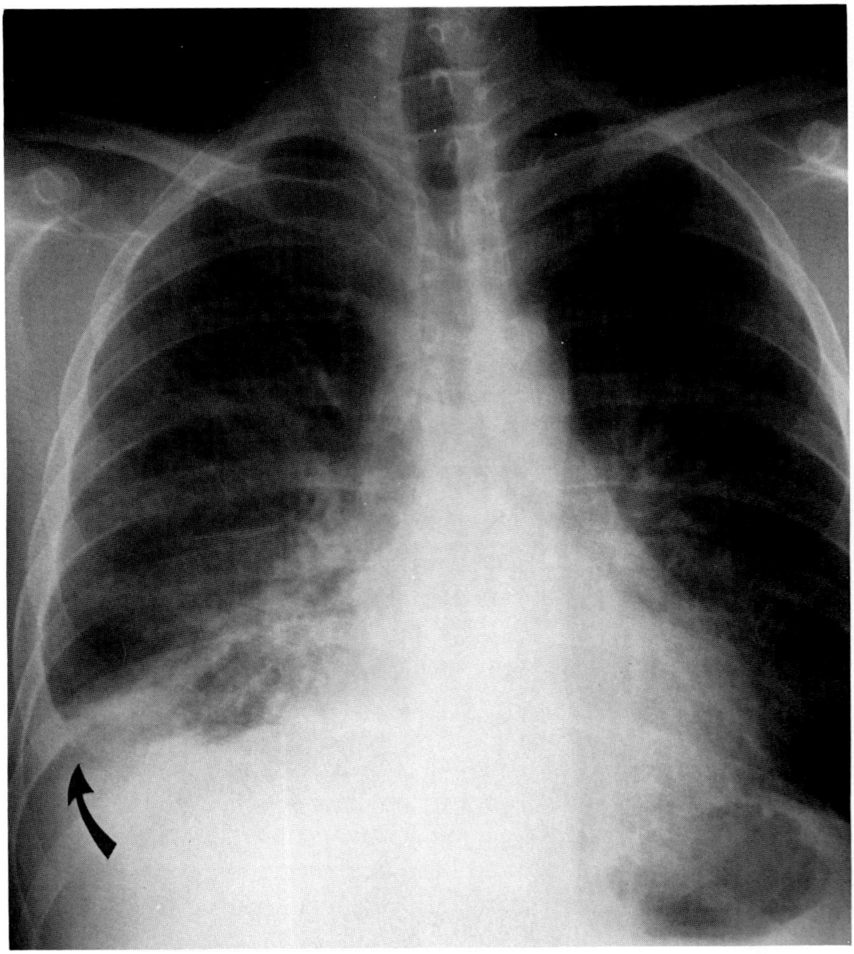

Figure 22A Lung Kaposi's sarcoma. Right pleural effusion (arrow) was biopsy positive for Kaposi's sarcoma in this patient with perihilar infiltrates of *Pneumocystis carinii* pneumonia.

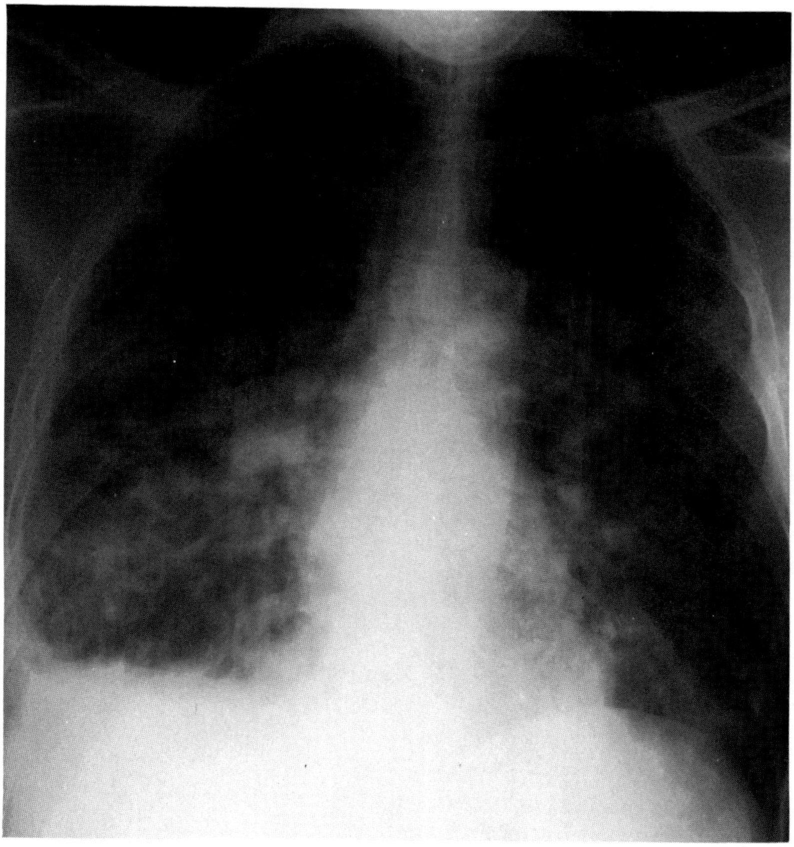

Figure 22B Parenchymal nodules of Kaposi's sarcoma developed with further progression of disease (autopsy proven). (Courtesy of Philip C. Goodman, M.D.)

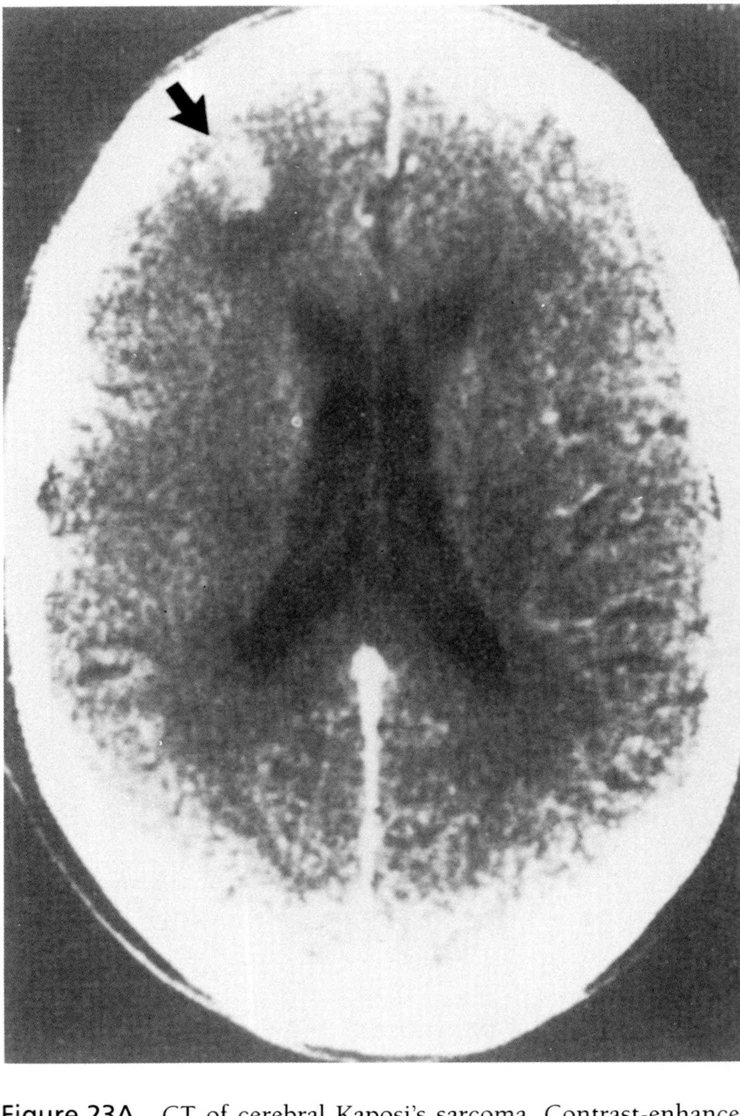

Figure 23A CT of cerebral Kaposi's sarcoma. Contrast-enhanced CT scan of the brain demonstrates focal lesion of Kaposi's sarcoma (arrow), which is homogeneously hyperdense and has little surrounding edema and little mass effect.

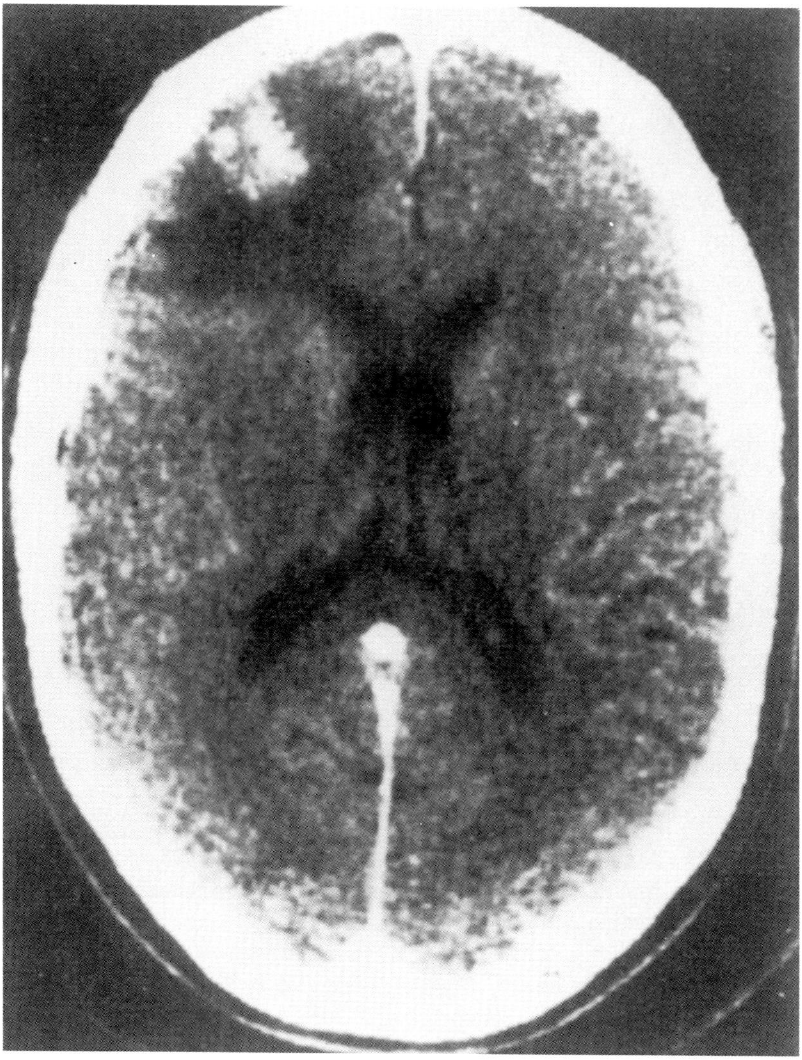

Figure 23B Reimaging 3 months later demonstrates progression in the size of the lesion despite interval radiation treatment with 3000 rad (30 Gy) (Kaposi's sarcoma proven at autopsy). (Reproduced from Reference 34 with permission.)

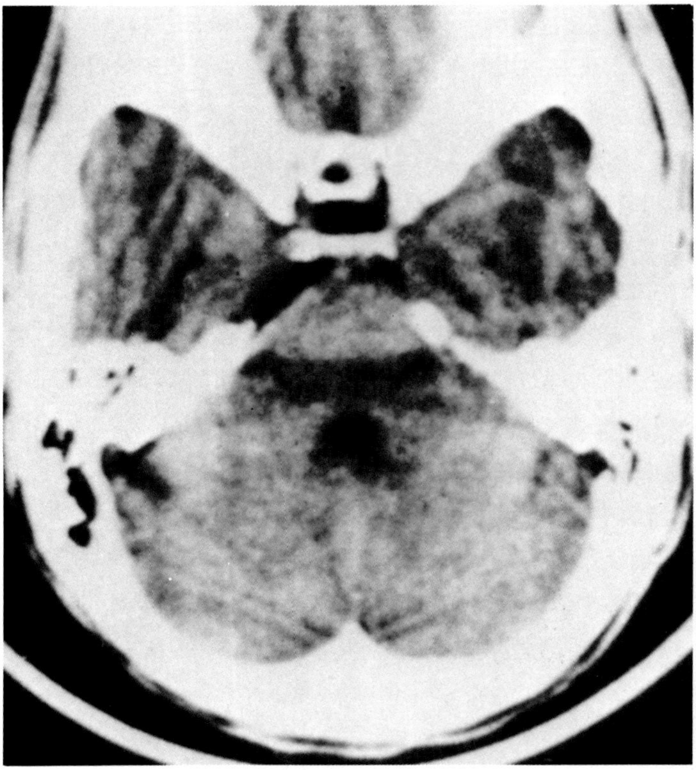

A

Figure 24 Magnetic resonance of cerebral Kaposi's sarcoma. Noncontrast CT scan (A) of the posterior fossa fails to demonstrate focal lesion of Kaposi's sarcoma, which is seen on magnetic resonance image (B) as an area of abnormal high-intensity signal (arrow) posterolateral to the fourth ventricle (spin echo image, TR = 1.5 sec, TE = 105 msec) (autopsy-proven Kaposi's sarcoma). (Reproduced from Reference 35 with permission.)

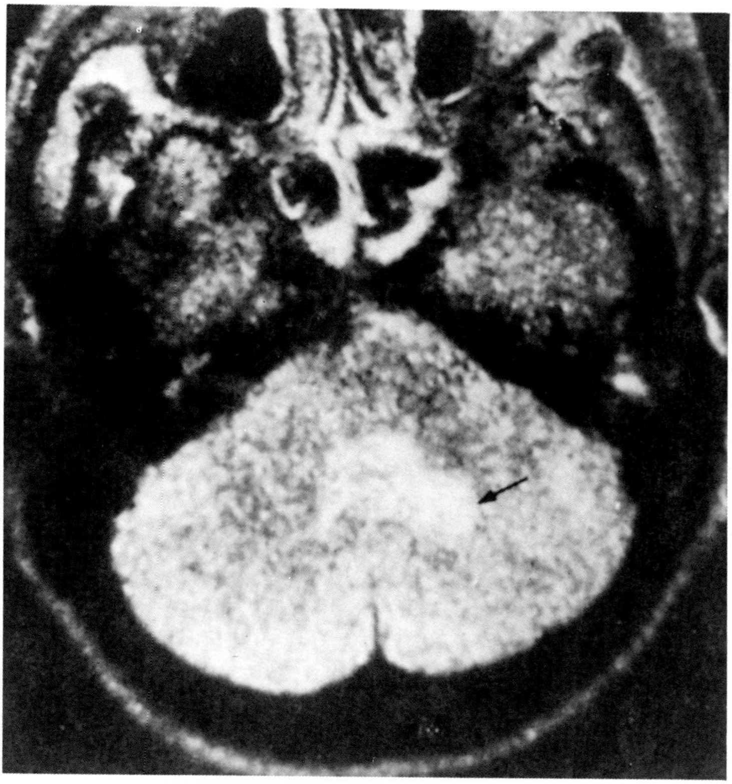

Figure 24B

lymphoma in patients with AIDS is that of a hypodense lesion on a noncontrast scan that demonstrates irregular enhancement (increased density) after intravenous contrast administration, often in a nodular or ringlike pattern (35). Surrounding edema may be prominent, and multifocal lesions are common.

Comparison of the abilities of computed tomography and magnetic resonance in detecting and evaluating central nervous system disease in neurologically symptomatic patients with AIDS has demonstrated differing advantages of each modality (35). High-resolution CT with intravenous contrast enhancement is superior to magnetic resonance for differentiating a lesion from surrounding edema, discriminating between lesions in close proximity, locating lesions for biopsy, judging lesion activity, detecting small cortical lesions with minimal edema, and spatial resolution. Magnetic resonance is superior to CT in evaluating white-matter lesions and detecting small lesions surrounded by edema. Magnetic resonance demonstrates greater contrast resolution and, overall, is more sensitive than CT in the detection of focal mass lesions. However, the preferred modality for the detection and characterization of intracerebral Kaposi's sarcoma must await further experience with each technique.

REFERENCES

1. Reeder M. Kaposi's sarcoma. In: Radiology of Tropical Diseases. Baltimore, William & Wilkins, 1981; 889–908.
2. Palmer PES. The radiological changes of Kaposi's sarcoma. ACTA 1962; XVIII:87–99.
3. Taylor JF, Templeton AC, Vogel CL, Ziegler JL, Kyalwazi SK. Kaposi's sarcoma in Uganda: a clinico-pathological study. Int J Cancer 1971; 8:122–35.
4. Baddeley H, Bhana D. Lymphography in Kaposi's sarcoma. Clin Radiol 1971; 22:391–400.
5. Friedman SL, Wright TL, Altman DF. Gastrointestinal Kaposi's sarcoma in patients with acquired immunodeficiency syndrome: endoscopic and autopsy finding. Gastroenterology 1985; 1:102–8.

6. Safai B, Johnson KG, Myskowski PL, et al. The natural history of Kaposi's sarcoma in the acquired immunodeficiency syndrome. Ann Intern Med 1985; 103:744–50.
7. Wall SD, Friedman SL, Margulis AR. Gastrointestinal Kaposi's sarcoma in AIDS: radiographic manifestations. J Clin Gastroenterol 1984; 6:165–71.
8. Rose HS, Balthazar EJ, Megibow AJ, Horowitz L, Laubenstein LJ. Alimentary tract involvement in Kaposi's sarcoma: radiographic and endoscopic findings in 25 homosexual men. AJR 1982; 139:661–6.
9. Wall SD, Ominsky S, Altman DF, Perkins CL, Sollitto R, Goldberg HI, Margulis AR. Multifocal abnormalities of the gastrointestinal tract in AIDS. AJR 1986; 146:1–5.
10. Hill CA, Harle TS, Mansell PWA. The prodrome, Kaposi's sarcoma and infections associated with acquired immunodeficiency syndrome: radiologic findings in 39 patients. Radiology 1983; 149:393–9.
11. Radin DR, Fong TL, Halls JM, Pontrelli GN. Monilial enteritis in acquired immunodeficiency syndrome. AJR 1983; 141:1289–90.
12. Balthazar EJ, Megibow AJ, Hulnick DH. Cytomegalovirus esphagitis and gastritis in AIDS. AJR 1985; 144:1201–4.
13. Bern RN, Wall SD, McArdle CB, McCutchan JA, Clemett AR, Rosenblum JS, Premkumer A, Megibow AJ. Cryptosporidiosis of the stomach and small intestine in patients with AIDS. AJR 1984; 143:549–54.
14. Wall SD. Abdominal radiology of acquired immunodeficiency syndrome. Contemp Diag Radiol 1986; 9(20):1–6.
15. Emery C, Wall SD, Federle MP, Sooy D. Pharyngeal Kaposi's sarcoma in acquired immunodeficiency syndrome. AJR 1986; 147: 919–922.
16. Ziegler JL, Beckstead JA, Volberding PA, et al. Non-Hodgkin's lymphoma in 90 homosexual men: relation to generalized lymphadenopathy and the acquired immunodeficiency syndrome. N Engl J Med 1984; 311:565–70.
17. Moon KL Jr, Federle MP, Abrams DI, Volberding P, Lewis BJ. Kaposi's sarcoma and lymphadenopathy syndrome: limitations of abdominal CT in acquired immunodeficiency syndrome. Radiology 1984; 150:479–83.
18. Jeffrey RB Jr, Nyberg DA, Bottle K, Abrams DI, Federle MP, Wall SD, Wing VW, Laing FC. Abdominal CT in acquired immunodeficiency syndrome. AJR 1986; 146:7–13.

19. Sider L, Mintzer RA, Mendlson EB, Rogers LF, Degesys GE. Radiographic findings in infectious proctitis in homosexual men. AJR 1982; 139:667–71.
20. Nyberg DA, Federle MP, Jeffrey RB, Bottles K, Wofsy CB. Abdominal CT findings of disseminated *Mycobacterium avium-intracellulare* in AIDS. AJR 1985; 145:297–9.
21. Strom RL, Greenings RP. AIDS with *Mycobacterium avium-intracellulare* lesions resembling those of Whipple's disease. N Engl J Med 1983; 309:1323–4.
22. Roth RI, Owen RL, Keven DF. AIDS with *Mycobacterium avium-intracellulare* lesions resembling those of Whipple's disease. N Engl J Med 1983; 309:1324–5.
23. Vincent ME, Robbins AH. *Mycobacterium avium-intracellulare* complex enteritis: pseudo-Whipple's disease in AIDS. AJR 1985; 144:921–2.
24. McGauley DI, Naidich DP, Leitman BS, Reede DL, Laubenstein L. Radiographic patterns of opportunistic lung infections and Kaposi sarcoma in homosexual men. AJR. 1982; 139:653–8.
25. Cohen BA, Pomeranz S, Rabinowitz JG, Rosen MJ, Train JS, Norton KI, Mendelson DS. Pulmonary complications of AIDS: radiologic features. AJR 1984; 143:115–22.
26. Epstein DM, Gefter WB, Conrad K, Kelley MA, Miller WT. Lung disease in homosexual men. Diag Radiol 1982; 143(1):7–10.
27. Kornfeld H, Axelrod JL. Pulmonary presentation of Kaposi's sarcoma in a homosexual patient. Ann Rev Respir Dis 1983; 127:248–9.
28. Kaplan LD, Hopewell PC, Jaffe H, Goodman PC, Bottles K, Volberding PA. Kaposi's sarcoma involving the lung in patients with the acquired immunodeficiency syndrome. AIDS Res (in press).
29. Brown RKJ, Huberman RP, Gregory V. Pulmonary features of Kaposi's sarcoma. AJR 1982; 139:659–60.
30. Stern RG, Gamsu G, Golden JA, Hirji M, Webb WR, Abrams DI. Intrathoracic adenopathy: differential features of AIDS and diffuse lymphadenopathy syndrome. AJR 1984; 142:689–92.
31. Fraser RG, Pare JAP. Diagnosis of Disease of the Chest. Philadelphia, WB Saunders, 1978:856–60.
32. Doppman JL, Geelhoed GW, Devita VT. Atypical radiographic features in *Pneumocystis carinii* pneumonia. Radiology 1975; 114:39–44.

33. Forrest JV. Radiographic findings in *Pneumocystis carinii* pneumonia. Radiology 1972; 103:539–44.
34. Kelley WM, Brant-Zawadzki M. Acquired immunodeficiency syndrome: neuroradiologic findings. Radiology 1983; 149:485–91.
35. Post MJD, Sheldon JJ, Hensley G, Soila K, Tobias JA, Chan JC, Quencer RM, Moskowitz LB. Central nervous system disease in acquired immunodeficiency syndrome: prospective correlation using CT, MR imaging, and pathologic studies. Radiology 1986; 158:141–8.

9

Radiation Therapy for Kaposi's Sarcoma in AIDS

John W. Harris*
Anthony M. Berson
Teri A. Reed†
William M. Wara
University of California
San Francisco, California

Current affiliations:
*St. Joseph Hospital, Eureka, California.
†Loyola University of Chicago, Stritch School of Medicine, Maywood, Illinois.

A substantial proportion of acquired immunodeficiency syndrome (AIDS) patients present with or later develop Kaposi's sarcoma. These tumors are histologically identical to the Kaposi's sarcoma seen in elderly males or in transplant patients (1,2), but their clinical course is usually far more aggressive. In some AIDS patients, Kaposi's sarcoma may represent no more than a minor problem, requiring no specific therapy. In others, however, many of the tumors cause serious cosmetic and functional difficulties. Kaposi's sarcoma in such patients is protean in its presentation and commonly causes psychological distress (e.g., cosmetically deforming skin lesions), pain, edema, visual difficulties, nutritional problems (e.g., with oral cavity or pharyngeal lesions), bleeding, and a variety of other clinical problems.

The treatment of Kaposi's sarcoma in patients with AIDS poses a difficult problem. Responses are sometimes obtained with chemotherapy or immunotherapy, but many patients cannot tolerate these systemic therapies or fail to respond to them. In some circumstances (e.g., a symptomatic oral cavity lesion), the use of local therapy is preferred. Indeed, it has been our experience that the majority of AIDS patients with Kaposi's sarcoma will sooner or later require irradiation for medical and psychological problems caused by their tumors.

Beginning in March 1983, we at the University of California–San Francisco (3) and colleagues at New York University (4,5) and Memorial-Sloan Kettering (6) began to treat AIDS patients who had Kaposi's sarcoma with radiation therapy. In this review, we will briefly survey the literature regarding the use of radiation therapy for "traditional" (or nonepidemic) Kaposi's sarcoma, as well as the more recent experience with the epidemic form of the tumor. We shall distill the currently available data and our own clinical experience in order to provide the clinician with specific guidelines for effective treatment of epidemic Kaposi's sarcoma in its more common clinical manifestations.

RADIATION THERAPY IN NONEPIDEMIC KAPOSI'S SARCOMA

It has long been known that moderate doses of ionizing radiation can affect permanent control of nonepidemic Kaposi's sarcoma, both in its traditional forms (7) and in immunosuppressed transplant patients (8). These data were analyzed by Cohen (7,9) and by Harwood (8) and were summarized recently by Harris and Reed (3). The conclusion was that nonepidemic Kaposi's sarcoma is controlled permanently (cured) by dose-fractionation schedules ranging from single doses of 600–800 cGy to multidose schemes up to 3000–4000 cGy in 150–300 cGy fractions. These regimens, applied with due regard to anatomic site and to technical factors (e.g., type of beam and use of bolus), result in cure rates exceeding 90%. Treatment-related side effects are rare, being limited to soft tissue necrosis in a few patients treated with large orthovoltage fields (3).

RADIATION THERAPY IN EPIDEMIC KAPOSI'S SARCOMA

In view of the efficacy of radiation therapy in nonepidemic Kaposi's sarcoma, it was anticipated that the epidemic form of the tumor would also be radiosensitive. Initially, AIDS patients with Kaposi's sarcoma were treated with a variety of radiation dose-fractionation regimens that were based on the experience with nonepidemic tumors and deemed appropriate for specific clinical situations (Figure 1). It was immediately apparent that epidemic Kaposi's sarcoma usually responded well to radiation, but some unexpected results were encountered. Side effects were unusually severe at certain sites (e.g., oral mucosa), and a significant proportion of "successfully treated" patients eventually relapsed in the treated area. These observations, detailed below, led us to modify some of our original treatment strategies.

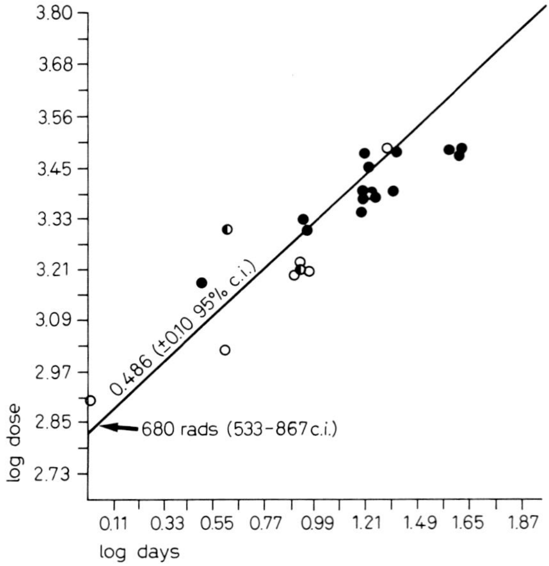

Figure 1 Regression analysis of all published literature for control of classic Kaposi's sarcoma and comparison with immunosuppressed renal transplant patients (○, ◐) and with (●) AIDS patients (UCSF data). The half-filled symbols represent patients in whom treatment failed. The regression line has a slope of 0.486 ± 0.100 (95% confidence interval) and an intercept of 2.832 ± 0.106 (95% confidence interval), the latter corresponding to a single dose of 680 (533–867) rad. (From Reference 3.)

Review of Published Data

The first reports of radiotherapy of AIDS-associated Kaposi's sarcoma, by Cooper et al. (5), Harris and Reed (3), and Nisce and Safai (6), all noted remarkably similar results. Although limited to small numbers of patients and relatively short follow-up times, these reports indicated that epidemic Kaposi's sarcoma was indeed sensitive to radiation therapy and that, with certain exceptions, doses similar to those used for nonepidemic Kaposi's sarcoma seemed adequate. Tumors of the eyelid and lymph nodes appeared to require higher doses than cutaneous or mucosal lesions (see below), but there was evidence that even Kaposi's sarcoma involving lung (10) and other organs could be treated effectively. The recommendations that emerged from these analyses ranged from weekly whole-body electron beam therapy (11) to focal x-ray treatments at single doses of 800 cGy to fractionated doses up to 4500 cGy in 4–5 weeks.

This early experience also revealed that although small skin lesions could be treated without side effects, some other areas of the body seemed unusually sensitive and required the use of low dose fractions. The oral cavity, for example, proved particularly sensitive in AIDS patients. Of our first 28 patients, 6 suffered severe mucositis that required intensive supportive care and even hospitalization. These mucosal reactions were often seen with doses as low as 1200 cGy, even with low dose fractionation. This experience has caused us and others to treat Kaposi's sarcoma in the oropharynx-hypopharynx carefully and to use pretreatment prophylaxis with appropriate antifungal and antiviral agents.

Similarly, treatment of large volumes in the presence of lymphedema produced toxic skin reactions in 20% of patients so treated that were far more severe than would have been anticipated. Of our first 45 patients, 5 (11%) developed pain, erythema, and edema suggestive of cellulitis; all responded to antibiotics, although no organisms could be cultured.

These observations have led us to modify our treatment techniques and to alter our expectations of efficacy for some disease sites. With longer follow-up, we began to see recurrences within previously treated volumes that required retreatment. Moreover, we and others (12) began to observe unusually severe toxicity in some patients who were receiving concomitant chemotherapy and/or immunotherapy; this, too, led to altered treatment policies. These observations are summarized in the next section.

Update of Published Data

One of the first observations that emerged with extended follow-up was that although palliation was achieved in about 90% of patients who were treated for symptoms (measured at 3–6 months post-treatment), recurrences became evident after 6 months in patients who survived this long. By 1 year postradiation, the rate of local control decreased to 67% (12 of 18 patients), and by 18 months only 50% of surviving patients (3 of 6) had no evidence of disease at the treated site.

We attempted retrospectively to correlate palliation rate and duration of response with doses and fractionation schedules used, particularly with respect to the use of single-dose (800 cGy) treatment versus fractionated treatment. As indicated above, failure rates at 6 months were about 10% with the fractionated regimens (and 33% at 1 year), whereas with single doses (800 cGy), 10 of 14 patients (73%) for whom follow-up was available required retreatment for recurrence within this time frame. This suggests that whereas single-dose treatment is highly effective for palliation and may be particularly useful in symptomatic patients with a limited life expectancy, it is not the treatment of choice for patients with longer life expectancy. We must emphasize, however, that this conclusion is a preliminary one based on retrospective analysis; a randomized trial, such as that being mounted by the Radiation Treatment Oncology Group, will be required to definitively answer the question.

Finally, treatment related complications continue to concern us. We and others (13) recognized very early the unusual radiosensitivity of the oral mucosa in AIDS patients, and this has continued to impress us. Even with the use of prophylaxis with topical antifungal and antiviral agents, we still see impressive mucositis in some patients at doses as low as 1200 cGy. Accordingly, we usually treat head and neck fields slowly (e.g., 140–160 cGy/day or less) and observe the patient carefully, interrupting treatment at the first sign of significant or symptomatic mucositis. Adverse reactions, both mucosal and cutaneous, appear to be particularly common in patients who are on or have recently been on chemotherapy and perhaps immunotherapy (12). We attempt to avoid such concomitant treatment.

Treatment Recommendations by Site

Cutaneous Lesions

In treating skin lesions for cosmetic reasons, we have found that superficial, nodular lesions are more responsive than flat, diffuse lesions. Only a small percentage of patients have complete disappearance of the lesion; these tend to be of the nodular variety. Results are better when bolus (e.g., wax or a wet towel) is used with photon energies greater than orthovoltage or when electrons are available. Radiation therapy has been extremely successful in controlling the pain associated with Kaposi's sarcoma lesions, but we have had variable success when treating skin lesions that are associated with edema. Although these latter lesions usually respond, the edema does not always resolve completely. In contrast, edema due to vascular or lymphatic obstruction will resolve if the source of obstruction is treated.

At present we usually treat cutaneous lesions with one of three daily fractionation schemes: 200 cGy per fraction to a total dose of 2000–3000 cGy, 400 cGy per fraction to a total of 2000–2400 cGy, or 800 cGy in a single fraction. We use the smaller fractions as the treatment volume increases. The single fraction is used less frequently now because the time to relapse appears to be shorter than with conventional fractionation (see Table 1). The soles and palms tend to be much more sensitive to radiation, and it is not unusual to see severe skin reactions in these areas. The use of appropriate antibiotics for cellulitis should be considered in such cases.

Mucosal Lesions

The oral mucosa in patients with AIDS is exquisitely sensitive to radiation. We have abandoned our early practice of using 400 cGy

Table 1 Duration of Response in Patients Treated with a Single Fraction of 800 cGy (March–October 1985)

Site	No. treated	Mean time to relapse (months)	Range
Feet	7	5.3	3–9
Toes	3	8	5–11
Nose	2	2	1–3
Penis	2	11	10–12
Extremity	5	7.6	5–12

fractions to a total dose of 2400 cGy and now recommend daily fractions as low as 150 cGy to total doses of about 1500–2000 cGy. We have delivered higher total doses to those patients who experienced moderate side effects or whose tumors showed slow response, but it is not yet clear that a dose-response relationship exists. We attempt to minimize the severity of the mucositis by the use of medication (antifungal troches for 3 days prior to radiotherapy and daily for the duration of treatments) and by withholding concomitant chemotherapy or immunotherapy whenever possible.

We have treated a few patients with Kaposi's sarcoma of the gastrointestinal tract who had generally far advanced disease. In most cases good symptomatic responses were achieved with relatively low doses (e.g., 1200–1600 cGy in three or four fractions).

Kaposi's Sarcoma in Lymph Nodes

Many patients with AIDS have either benign lymphoid hyperplasia or actual Kaposi's sarcoma involvement of the lymph node system. It is the latter that responds to radiotherapy. Inguinal and cervical nodes are commonly affected. We have had good success in palliating the pain and deformity associated with lymphadenopathy in noninguinal sites. Of patients treated for nodal disease in these sites, 82% have had durable responses (minimum follow-up of 6 months) with 800 cGy in one fraction or 2000 cGy in ten fractions. In contrast, we have achieved only a 61% response rate in patients whose inguinal nodes were treated. In retrospect, many of these patients may have had pelvic as well as inguinal node involvement (with the entire area therefore not included in the treatment field), and many probably had very bulky disease requiring higher doses. We now obtain a CT scan of the abdomen and pelvis to evaluate patients who present with lower extremity edema and design our treatment fields using this information.

Eye and Eyelid

Kaposi's sarcoma lesions may involve the eye, either on the eyelid or on the conjunctival surface itself. These lesions can cause impairment of vision directly or secondarily by causing ptosis or profound edema of the soft tissues surrounding the orbit. We recommend doses around 3000 cGy using conventional fractionation in treating these lesions. Superior results have been noted with this regimen compared with 2000 cGy, in which a 32% local failure rate within 6 months was obtained.

Lung

At the UCSF we have treated two patients with Kaposi's sarcoma of the lung, both presenting with marked dyspnea and hemoptysis. Both patients received 900 cGy in six fractions to the whole lung, and both had marked improvement in their symptoms without acute side effects. The first patient died of *Pneumocystis carinii* pneumonia 3 months after treatment; the second is still alive at 6 months. Other authors have had a similar experience (10). The total dose to both lungs should be limited to 1500 cGy in 150 cGy fractions, and prophylactic antibiotic therapy for *P. carinii* pneumonia should be considered, depending on the clinical situation.

PRACTICAL ASPECTS OF TREATMENT

Treatment Procedures

We have generally followed the recommendations of the U.S. Department of Health and Human Services (HHS) and the Centers for Disease Control (CDC) with respect to protection of health care workers and handling of equipment used to treat AIDS patients. We prefer not to tattoo these patients but have done so on occasion when the treatment setup was complicated (especially head and neck sites) or when the anticipated duration of treatments was long. In these circumstances the needles used are disposed of directly as recommended by the HHS (14). Gloves are worn by the personnel involved. Bite blocks (used for head and neck treatments) are stored separately and covered. The recommendation of the CDC is for these to be rinsed after each treatment in a solution of 5% bleach (15). Bite blocks are disposed of at completion of treatment, and the metal base is then sterilized. Eye shields, used infrequently, are handled in a similar way. The treatment table is cleansed with a solution of bleach after each AIDS patient is treated. The water bath we use as bolus for treating lesions of the feet is also cleaned with a bleach solution.

Blood counts should be monitored frequently when large fields are being treated. Most AIDS patients have low baseline counts, and it is not unusual to see decreases in leukocyte counts, especially in patients who receive other marrow-toxic therapies.

Coordination and In-service Training

In-service training is given periodically to the personnel involved in treating AIDS patients. The radiologic technologists and nurses are kept up to date with CDC recommended precautions. Because of the number of AIDS patients we have treated, a comfortable rapport has been established between medical personnel and patients. Many of our patients are referred from the AIDS clinic at San Francisco General Hospital, and a close working relationship exists with the staff of the AIDS clinic.

SUMMARY AND CONCLUSIONS

The treatment of Kaposi's sarcoma in AIDS patients is a therapeutic challenge. The combination of a relatively rare tumor in a fragile host with unexpected treatment-related morbidity has caused progress in therapy to be slow. Because of the relative uniqueness of the clinical setting surrounding each AIDS patient, it has been difficult to establish rigorous studies to evaluate effective total doses and optimal fractionation regimens. Short life span following diagnosis, opportunistic infections, and other therapies have obscured results. Varying social support structures for each patient have made acceptance of treatment, compliance, and follow-up difficult in some cases. Until a cure or prevention is found, radiation therapy will continue to play a prominent palliative role. Our goal is to offer a treatment that can be delivered over a relatively short period of time, that has low morbidity, and that has an acceptable duration of response. Each treatment therefore needs to be individualized based on the clinical setting. We have tried not to present a "cookbook" of treatment regimens, but rather observations and recommendations based on our experience. Our results and conclusions concur generally with the recently published series from New York City (16). We will continue to pursue new dose-fractionation studies, management policies for side effects, and new treatments, including radiolabeled antibody therapy.

REFERENCES

1. Friedman-Kien AE, Laubenstein LJ, Rubinstein P, et al. Disseminated Kaposi's sarcoma in homosexual men. Ann Intern Med 1982; 96(1):693–700.
2. Gottlieb G, Ackerman AB. Kaposi's sarcoma. An extensively disseminated form in young homosexual men. Hum Pathol 1982; 13:882–92.
3. Harris JW, Reed TA. Kaposi's sarcoma in AIDS: the role of radiation therapy. Front Radiat Ther Oncol 1985; 19:126–32.
4. Cooper JS, Fried PR. Defining the role of radiation therapy in the

management of epidemic Kaposi's sarcoma (abstract). ASTRO (1985).
5. Cooper JS, Fried PR, Lansenstein LJ. Initial observations of the effect of radiotherapy on epidemic Kaposi's sarcoma. JAMA 1985; 252 (7):934–5.
6. Nisce LZ, Safai B. Radiation therapy of Kaposi's sarcoma in AIDS: Memorial Sloan-Kettering experience. Front Radiat Ther Oncol 1985; 19:133–7.
7. Cohen L, et al. Treatment of Kaposi's sarcoma by radiation. Acta Union Int Contre Cancrum 1962; 18:502–9.
8. Harwood AR, Osoba D, Hofstader SL, et al. Kaposi's sarcoma in recipients of renal transplants. Am J Med 1979; 67:759–65.
9. Cohen L. Dose, time and volume parameters in irradiation therapy and Kaposi's sarcoma. Br J Radiol 1962; 35:484–8.
10. Nobler MP. Pulmonary irradiation for Kaposi's sarcoma in AIDS. Am J Clin Oncol 1985; 8(5):441–4.
11. Nisce LZ, et al. Once weekly total and subtotal skin electron beam therapy for Kaposi's sarcoma. Cancer 1981; 47:640–4.
12. Real RF, Krown SE, Nisce LZ, Oettgen HF. Unexpected toxicity from radiation therapy in two patients with Kaposi's sarcoma receiving interferon. J Biol Response Mod 1985; 4(2):141–6.
13. Grepp DR, Chandler W, Hyams V. Primary Kaposi's sarcoma of the head and neck. Ann Intern Med 1984; 100:107–14.
14. MMWR, November 5, 1982; 31(43):577–80.
15. MMWR, November 15, 1985; 34(45):681–95.
16. Nobler MP, Leddy ME, Huh SH. The impact of palliative irradiation on the management of patients with the acquired immune deficiency syndrome. J Clin Oncol 1986; 5:107–12.

10

Chemotherapy

Paul A. Volberding
University of California
and San Francisco General Hospital
San Francisco, California

Kaposi's sarcoma occurs in 20–30% of homosexual men with the acquired immunodeficiency syndrome (AIDS) at the time of first AIDS diagnosis. It develops in many additional patients during the course of their disease and represents a significant clinical management problem. Although not often directly the cause of death, it can contribute to the morbidity of the disease and, when present on exposed portions of the skin, contributes to the social isolation experienced by many AIDS patients. For these reasons, control of this malignancy is an important goal of AIDS patient management. Radiation therapy (see Chapter 9) has shown activity in controlling local disease (1,2), but the multicentric nature of this tumor often dictates the need for systemic approaches. Of these, chemotherapy with cytotoxic agents and biologic approaches with recombinant α-interferon have been shown to be active. This chapter briefly reviews the background of chemotherapy in non-AIDS-related Kaposi's sarcoma and then discusses the various agents that have been used in patients with AIDS. Finally, we offer management guidelines to help in deciding which approach to recommend.

Unfortunately for the clinician interested in the management of AIDS-related Kaposi's sarcoma, there is very little reliable information regarding the chemotherapy of Kaposi's sarcoma in non-AIDS patients. In classic Kaposi's sarcoma in the elderly, therapy is not often required given the indolent nature of the disease. There have been occasional reports that chemotherapy, especially with vinblastine, is active in conventional doses (3–8,15).

In African Kaposi's sarcoma, investigations were conducted in the 1970s. Here a substantial, and in some cases striking, activity for a variety of chemotherapeutic agents was found (3,9–15). Response rates of >90% were reported, for example with vinblastine, vincristine, bleomycin, actinomycin D, and others (Table 1). Survival follow-up on these studies was often impossible, however, so the duration of responses has not been defined. Also, the relevance of these reports in African Kaposi's sarcoma to current cases in AIDS is debatable.

Chemotherapy of patients with Kaposi's sarcoma in the setting of renal transplantation has also been anecdotal (3,15). Agents such as vinblastine have been effective, but most of these patients

Table 1 Therapy of Kaposi's Sarcoma (Non-AIDS Related)

Risk group	Active agents	Comments
Elderly men (classic Kaposi's Sarcoma)	Vinblastine	Anecdotal reports and small series: some long remissions
Black Africans	Vincristine, vinblastine, bleomycin, actinomycin D, ICRF-159	Limited duration of follow-up and most studies uncontrolled; most active in nodular Kaposi's Sarcoma, least active in lymphadenopathic Kaposi's Sarcoma in children
Renal transplant recipients		Anecdotal reports; most benefit seen with discontinuation of immunosuppressive medications

Source: From References 3–15.

have been managed by discontinuation of their immunosuppressive medications (16–18).

A number of single-agent therapies and occasional combinations of cytotoxic agents have been attempted and reported in AIDS. This work is continuing, but already substantial activity has been reported for vinblastine, vincristine, etoposide, and recombinant α-interferon. The combination of adriamycin, bleomycin, and vinblastine has also been reported to be effective, but a number of single agents have been found not to have significant activity.

VINBLASTINE

Investigators, particularly in San Francisco, have used single-agent vinblastine on a weekly schedule for AIDS-related Kaposi's sarcoma (19). In a study in which patients were treated with all stages of Kaposi's sarcoma and with or without lymphoma-like B symptoms, vinblastine in an intravenous dose of 4–8 mg weekly resulted in an objective response rate of approximately 25%. Most responses were partial rather than complete, and the median duration of response was approximately 6 months.

Toxicity with single-agent vinblastine in AIDS-related Kaposi's sarcoma is minimal, with the drug primarily causing a reduction in granulocytes, which can be managed by vinblastine dosage adjustments. Careful immunologic studies have not been performed in this or in most other trials of chemotherapy agents, but the investigators were not suspicious that vinblastine was significantly immunotoxic as rates of opportunistic infections in treated patients appeared comparable to those for untreated AIDS patients.

VINCRISTINE

Vincristine has also been shown to be effective in AIDS-related Kaposi's sarcoma. In a study conducted at Memorial-Sloan Kettering, in patients with Kaposi's sarcoma who were also thrombocytopenic, a 75% objective response rate was reported (20). This report found a low incidence of neurotoxicity. In our own experience in San Francisco, however, a substantial incidence of peripheral neuropathies was observed when vincristine was used as a single agent. These issues will require clarification and confirmation with additional studies.

ETOPOSIDE (VP-16)

Etoposide was used in AIDS-related Kaposi's sarcoma in an important early study from New York University (21). Investigators there found a high response rate (>50%) using etoposide 150 mg/m^2 body surface area intravenously on 3 consecutive days every 3–4 weeks. In this study, patients were selected by the absence of systemic signs, making a direct comparison with studies of vinca alkaloids somewhat difficult. Etoposide in these studies and in subsequent work by other investigators causes only modest toxicity, although patients commonly experience alopecia. Hematologic toxicity was acceptable in which the drug primarily caused a decrease in granulocyte count. Etoposide is used by many clinicians as a first-line therapy for advanced Kaposi's sarcoma and as a second-line therapy after vinca alkaloids in patients with more minimal disease.

ALTERNATING VINBLASTINE AND VINCRISTINE

The combination of vinblastine and vincristine has also been explored in AIDS-related Kaposi's sarcoma. In studies recently reported, vinblastine was alternated with vincristine as a single agent weekly injected, using the dose for each drug as discussed above (22). This alternating regimen was chosen in an attempt to decrease toxicity, especially hematologic and neurologic toxicity, thereby permitting higher aggregate drug dosing. With this ap-

Table 2 Use of Alternating Vincristine and Vinblastine in AIDS-Related Kaposi's Sarcoma

Dose
Vincristine, 2.0 mg total dose, intravenous bolus
Vinblastine, 4–8 mg total dose, intravenous bolus
Schedule
Use above drugs as single agents weekly in alternating schedule
Adjusting for toxicity
Vincristine
For mild neuropathy decrease to 1.4 mg total dose
For moderate or severe neuropathy discontinue and use single-agent vinblastine
Vinblastine: Start at 4 mg and increase dose by 1 mg increments to maintain total WBC of 2.5–3000 cells/mm^3

proach, an objective response rate of 40% (again usually partial responses) was reported. Toxicity was minimal, primarily consisting of a modest decrement in granulocyte count and occasional peripheral neuropathy. At San Francisco General Hospital, this alternating regimen is our current first choice for patients with most stages of AIDS-related Kaposi's sarcoma, although other single-agent therapies are being explored (Table 2).

COMBINATION CHEMOTHERAPY

The combination of adriamycin, bleomycin, and vinblastine is the only cytotoxic combination therapy that has been explored in any detail in patients with AIDS-related Kaposi's sarcoma. Again in studies at New York University, this combination was reported early in the epidemic to have a substantial response rate (50–75%) (21,23). Many of these patients had rather advanced disease and/or the presence of systemic signs and symptoms. A problem with this combination was the apparent increase in the rate of opportunistic infections in patients receiving this combination. Although this was not a controlled study and has not been repeated, most clinicians are disinclined to recommend combination of cytotoxic agents except in far advanced stages or in patients with pulmonary Kaposi's sarcoma, which is known to be rapidly fatal.

α-INTERFERON

Recombinant human α-interferon has been used by several centers as experimental therapy for AIDS-related Kaposi's sarcoma. Generally, higher doses (≥20,000,000 units/m^2) have been required to achieve an objective response rate of about 40% in unselected patients with Kaposi's sarcoma (24–27). Response rates are somewhat higher if data are analyzed to include only patients who do not have systemic B symptoms. Toxicities with recombinant α-interferon are primarily subjective, consisting of a flulike syndrome. In addition, reversible elevations in transaminase and decreases in total granulocyte counts have been reported.

α-interferon is not yet approved for use in AIDS-related Kaposi's sarcoma, but interest in this therapy is increasing given the recent demonstration of in vitro activity against the human immunodeficiency virus (HIV) (28). Also, it is suspected that, in contrast to a more aggressive cytotoxic chemotherapy agent, α-interferon is less immunotoxic and may be less associated with the complicating, and often fatal, opportunistic infections.

Given the availability of mild chemotherapy approaches with minimal subjective toxicity, the role of α-interferon in the management of Kaposi's sarcoma has yet to be clearly defined. It does deserve a place in our armamentarium against this malignancy, however, and may be recommended early in the course of disease, particularly in patients without systemic symptoms.

MISCELLANEOUS AGENTS

A variety of other single agents have been explored and shown to be inactive. These include ICRF-159 (29), mitoxantrone (30), *cis*-retinoic acid (31), and vinzolidine. Agents under current investigation include methotrexate, bleomycin, and single-agent adriamycin.

RECOMMENDATIONS

Certainly the most pressing need is for a more accurate staging system for AIDS-related Kaposi's sarcoma. This would permit more rational subject section for clinical trials and would allow more adequate comparison of clinical trial results.

Single-agent cytotoxic drugs continue to deserve exploration. It is hoped that by adjusting doses and schedules more active and less immunotoxic regimens can be devised, perhaps moving to combination chemotherapy, as has been successful in other aggressive malignancies. There is, if anything, more hope in combinations of chemotherapy with biologic approaches, including antivirals, such as azidothymidine. This and other approaches will continue to make the therapy of Kaposi's sarcoma an active area of investigation in years to come. Meanwhile, the use of treatment guidelines, such as those shown in Table 3, are recommended.

Table 3 Guidelines for Therapy of AIDS-Related Kaposi's Sarcoma

Disease characteristics	First options	Second options
Minimal tumor extent,[a] slow rate of progression		
Favorable prognostic factors	No immediate treatment	Vinblastine-vincristine or α-IFN
Nonfavorable factors[b]	Vinblastine-vincristine or α-IFN	No immediate treatment
Extensive disease, rapid growth		
Favorable prognostic factors	Etoposide, adriamycin, vinca alkaloids	α-IFN
Unfavorable prognostic factors	Etoposide, adriamycin	Vinca alkaloids
Locally symptomatic lesions: lymphedema or painful necrotic lesions	Radiation therapy	

[a]Definitions vary; generally <25 cutaneous lesions, no known visceral involvement.
[b]Incompletely defined but include anemia, thrombocytopenia, leukopenia, elevated ESR, helper cell absolute number $\leq$ 100; systemic signs (fevers, weight loss, night sweats).

REFERENCES

1. Cooper J, Fried P, Laubenstein L. Initial observations of the effect of radiotherapy on epidemic Kaposi's sarcoma. JAMA 1984; 252:934–5.
2. Harris J, Reed T. Kaposi's sarcoma in acquired immune deficiency syndrome: the role of radiation therapy. Front Radiat Ther Oncol 1985; 19:126–32.
3. Odajnyk C, Muggia F. Treatment of Kaposi's sarcoma: overview and analysis by clinical setting. J Clin Oncol 1985; 3:1277–85.
4. Lanzotti V, Campos L, Sinkovics J, et al. Chemotherapy for advanced Kaposi's sarcoma. Arch Dermatol 1975; 111:1331–33.
5. Brambilla L, Boneschi V, Beretta G, Finzi A. Intralesional chemotherapy for Kaposi's sarcoma. Dermatologica 1984; 169:150.
6. Solan A, Greenwald E, Silvay O. Long-term complete remissions of Kaposi's sarcoma with vinblastine therapy. Cancer 1981; 47:637–9.
7. Tucker S, Winkelmann R. Treatment of Kaposi's sarcoma with vinblastine. Arch Dermatol 1976; 112:958–61.
8. Klein E, Schwartz R, Laor Y, et al. Treatment of Kaposi's sarcoma with vinblastine. Cancer 1980; 45:427–31.
9. Olweny C, Kaddumukasa A, Atine I, et al. Childhood Kaposi's sarcoma: clinical features and therapy. Cancer 1976; 33:555–60.
10. Kyalwazi S. Treatment of Kaposi's sarcoma. East Afr Med J August 1969; 450–8.
11. Olweny C, Toya T, Katongole-Mbidde E. Treatment of Kaposi's sarcoma by combination of actinomycin-D, vincristine and imidazole carboxamide (NSC-45388). Int J Cancer 1974; 14:649–56.
12. Vogel C, Primack A, Dhru D. Treatment of Kaposi's sarcoma with a combination of actinomycin-D and vincristine. Cancer 1973; 6:1382–9.
13. Vogel C, Templeton C, Templeton A, et al. Treatment of Kaposi's sarcoma with actinomycin-D and cyclophosphamide: results of a randomized clinical trial. Int J Cancer 1971; 8:136–43.
14. Olweny C, Masaba J, Sikyewunda W, Toya T. Treatment of Kaposi's sarcoma with ICRF-159 (NSC-129943). Cancer Treat Rep 1976; 60:111–3.
15. Volberding P, Conant M, Stricker R, Lewis B. Chemotherapy in advanced Kaposi's sarcoma. Implications for current cases in homosexual men. Am J Med 1983; 74:652–6.

16. Zisbrod Z, Haimov M, Schanzer H, et al. Kaposi's sarcoma after kidney transplantation. Report of complete remission of cutaneous and visceral involvement. Transplantation 1980; 30:383–4.
17. Stribling J, Weitzner S, Smith G. Kaposi's sarcoma in renal allograft recipients. Cancer 1978; 42:442–6.
18. Little P, Farthing C, Khader A, et al. Kaposi's sarcoma in a patient after renal transplantation. Postgrad Med J 1983; 59:325–6.
19. Volberding P, Abrams D, Conant M, et al. Vinblastine therapy for Kaposi's sarcoma in the acquired immune deficiency syndrome. Ann Intern Med 1985; 103:335–8.
20. Mintzer D, Real F, Jovino L, et al. Treatment of Kaposi's sarcoma and thrombocytopenia with vincristine in patients with acquired immune deficiency syndrome. Ann Intern Med 1985; 102:200–2.
21. Laubenstein L, Krigel R, Odajnyk C, et al. Treatment of epidemic Kaposi's sarcoma with etoposide or a combination of doxorubicin, bleomycin and vinblastine. J Clin Oncol 1984; 2:1115–20.
22. Kaplan L, Volberding P. Treatment of AIDS-related Kaposi's sarcoma with vincristine alternating with vinblastine. Cancer Treat Rep 1986; 70:1121–2.
23. Lewis B, Abrams D, Ziegler J. Single agent or combination chemotherapy of Kaposi's sarcoma in acquired immune deficiency syndrome. Am Soc Clin Oncol 1983; 2:59.
24. Groopman J, Gottlieb M, Goodman J. Recombinant alpha-2 interferon therapy of Kaposi's sarcoma associated with acquired immune deficiency syndrome. Ann Intern Med 1984; 100:671–6.
25. Gelmann E, Preble O, Steis R, et al. Human lymphoblastoid interferon treatment of Kaposi's sarcoma in the acquired immune deficiency syndrome. Clinical response and prognostic parameters. Am J Med 1985; 78:737–41.
26. Krown S, Real F, Vadhan-Raj S. Kaposi's sarcoma and the acquired immune deficiency syndrome treatment with recombinant interferon alpha and analysis of prognostic factors. Cancer 1986; 57: 1662.
27. Rios A, Mansell W, Newell G. Treatment of AIDS-related Kaposi's sarcoma with lymphoblastoid interferon. J Clin Oncol 1985; 3:506–12.
28. Volberding P, Mitsuyasu R. Recombinant interferon alpha in the treatment of acquired immune deficiency syndrome-related Kaposi's sarcoma. Semin Oncol 1985; 12:2–6.

29. Volberding P, Abrams D, Kaplan L, et al. Therapy of AIDS-related Kaposi's sarcoma with ICRF-159. Am Soc Clin Oncol 1985; 4:4.
30. Kaplan L, Volberding P. Failure (and danger) of mitozantrone in acquired immune deficiency syndrome related Kaposi's sarcoma (letter). Lancet 1985; 2:396.
31. Ziegler J, Volberding P, Itri L. Failure of isotretinoin in Kaposi's sarcoma. Lancet 1984; 2:641.

Index

About the Editors

John L. Ziegler is Associate Chief of Staff for Education at the Veterans Administration Medical Center and Professor of Medicine at the University of California, San Francisco. Previously he served as Director of the Uganda Cancer Institute at Makerere University Medical School in Kampala, Uganda (1967–72) and as Deputy Clinical Director of the National Cancer Institute in Bethesda, Maryland (1975–80). Dr. Ziegler was affiliated with the National Cancer Institute from 1966 to 1981, and was Editor-in-Chief of the *Journal of the National Cancer Institute* (1980–81). The author or co-author of over 170 articles, reviews, and book chapters as well as over 100 abstracts, he received the Albert and Mary Lasker Award in 1972 and the Heath Award of the M.D. Anderson Hospital and Tumor Institute in Houston, Texas in 1983. He is a member of the American Association for Cancer Research, American Federation for Clinical Research, American Society for Clinical Investigation, American Society of Clinical Oncology, and American Society of Hematology. Dr. Ziegler received the B.A. degree (1960) from Amherst College and M.D. degree (1964) from Cornell University Medical College.

Ronald F. Dorfman is Professor of Pathology and Co-Director of Surgical Pathology at Stanford University Medical Center in Stanford, California, where he has taught since 1968. Previously he taught at Washington University School of Medicine in St. Louis and served as a pathologist at the University of the Witwatersrand Medical School in Johannesburg, South Africa. The author or co-author of more than 120 articles and book chapters, he has co-edited two books, including *Malignant Lymphoma,* and he has given over 130 lectures and presentations throughout the world on Hodgkin's disease, malignant lymphomas, hematopathology, and Kaposi's sarcoma. Dr. Dorfman is an editorial board member of the journals *Cancer, Human Pathology,* and *Seminars in Diagnostic Pathology*. He is a member of the International Academy of Pathology, American Association of Pathologists, Arthur Purdy Stout Society of Surgical Pathologists, American Society of Hematology, and Society for Hematopathology, of which he was co-founder. Dr. Dorfman received the M.B. and B.Ch. degrees (1948) from the University of the Witwatersrand in Johannesburg, South Africa. In 1974 he gained membership in, and in 1980 was elected a Fellow of, the Royal College of Pathologists of England.